The
Estrogen Matters Diet

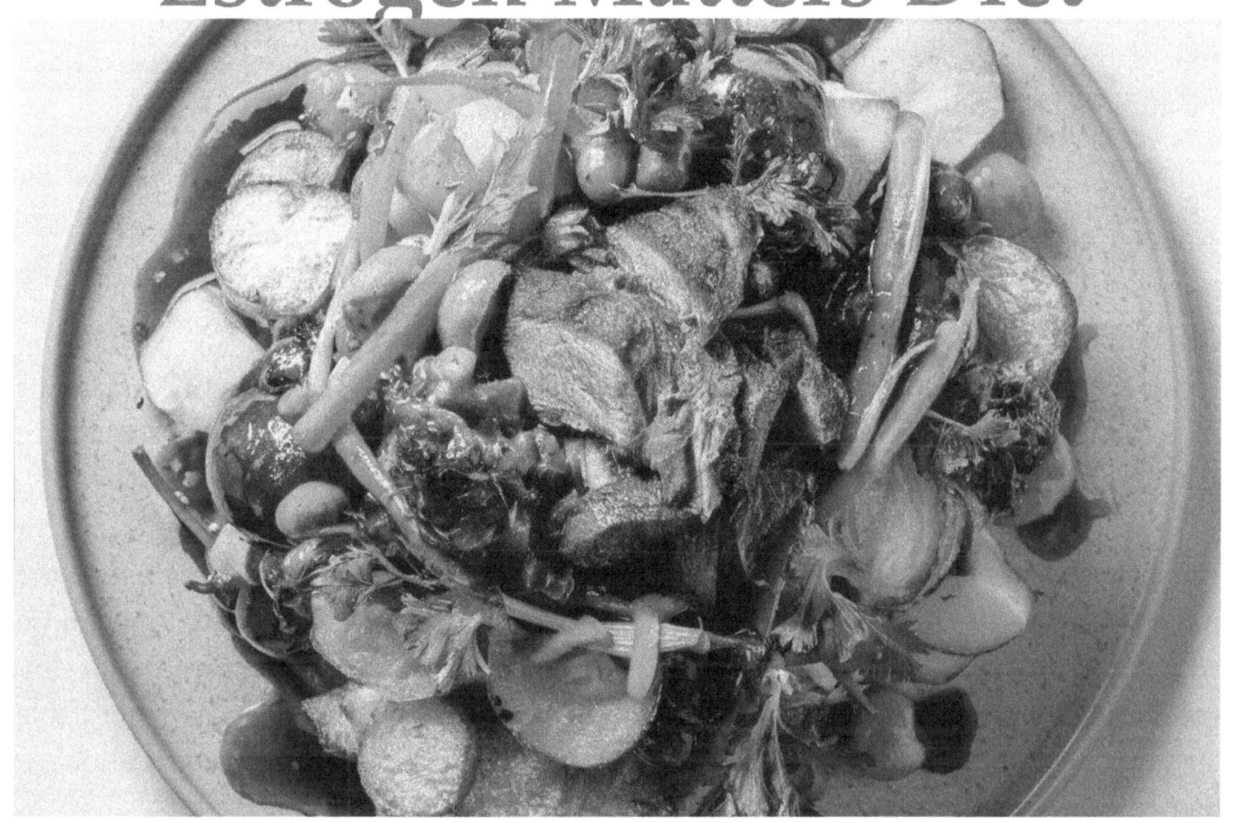

A Recipe Cookbook for Hormone-Balanced Health

Dr. Olivia Tastewell

Disclaimer:
This book is a work of [fiction/non-fiction]. Names, characters, places, and incidents either are products of the author's imagination or are used fictitiously. Any resemblance to actual persons, living or dead, events, or locales is entirely coincidental.

The information provided in this book is designed to provide helpful information on the subjects discussed. This book is not meant to be used, nor should it be used, to diagnose or treat any medical condition. The author and publisher are not responsible for any specific health or allergy needs that may require medical supervision and are not liable for any damages or negative consequences from any treatment, action, application, or preparation to any person reading or following the information in this book.

Table of content

CHAPTER 5: LUNCH RECIPES   51

CHAPTER 6: DINNER RECIPES   67

INTRODUCTION

AS WOMEN AGE, A HOST OF HEALTH REALITIES DEMAND ATTENTION AND proactive management. The transition through menopause brings significant hormonal changes that can profoundly impact your physical and emotional well-being. "The Estrogen Matters Diet: A Recipe Cookbook for Hormone-Balanced Health" offers a scientifically-grounded approach to support your body's evolving needs through targeted nutrition.

This introduction lays the foundation for understanding hormone replacement therapy (HRT), the critical role of estrogen in women's health, and how dietary choices can influence hormonal balance. Armed with this knowledge, you'll be better equipped to make informed decisions about your health and harness the power of nutrition to support your body's changing needs.

Hormone Replacement Therapy: Reexamining the Evidence

For years, hormone replacement therapy stood as a cornerstone in managing menopausal symptoms and promoting long-term health in women. However, its reputation suffered a significant setback in the early 2000s, leading many to abandon this once-celebrated treatment. To fully grasp the value of HRT, it's crucial to examine its history and the scientific evidence supporting its use.

The 1960s and 1970s saw researchers recognizing the potential benefits of replacing hormones lost during menopause. Initial studies yielded promising results, indicating that HRT could alleviate common menopausal symptoms such as hot flashes, night sweats, and vaginal dryness. Furthermore, long-term studies suggested potential protective effects against osteoporosis, cardiovascular disease, and cognitive decline. A dramatic shift occurred in 2002 with the publication of results from the Women's Health Initiative (WHI) study. This large-scale clinical trial reported an increased risk of breast cancer and cardiovascular events among women using a specific combination of hormones. The ensuing media coverage led to a sharp decline in HRT use, with many healthcare providers and patients alike avoiding the treatment. Subsequent analysis of the WHI data and numerous follow-up studies have revealed a more nuanced picture.

Current understanding indicates that the risks and benefits of HRT vary depending on factors such as a woman's age, time since menopause onset, and the specific hormones used. For many women, especially those under 60 or within 10 years of menopause onset, the benefits of HRT may indeed outweigh the risks.

Recent research has illuminated the potential protective effects of estrogen on various body systems. Estrogen plays a crucial role in maintaining bone density, potentially reducing the risk of osteoporosis and fractures. It also appears to have cardioprotective effects, particularly when initiated early in menopause. Some studies suggest that estrogen may even offer neuroprotective benefits, potentially reducing the risk of Alzheimer's disease and other forms of dementia.

As you consider your own health strategy, it's essential to approach HRT with a clear understanding of current research. Consult with a healthcare provider well-versed in up-to-date HRT studies to determine if this treatment option aligns with your individual health profile and goals.

Estrogen: A Powerful Force in Your Body

Estrogen, often labeled the "female hormone," exerts a far more complex and wide-ranging influence on your body than its name suggests. This potent hormone affects nearly every tissue and organ system, orchestrating a delicate balance that impacts your physical, emotional, and cognitive health.

At its core, estrogen comprises a group of hormones, with three main types found in your body: estradiol, estriol, and estrone. Estradiol, the most potent form, dominates during your reproductive years. As menopause approaches, estrone becomes more prominent, while estriol plays a significant role during pregnancy.

Your ovaries serve as the primary production site for estrogen, although smaller amounts are also synthesized in your adrenal glands, fat tissue, and brain. This hormone exerts its influence by binding to estrogen receptors distributed throughout your body, triggering a cascade of cellular responses.

In the reproductive system, estrogen regulates the menstrual cycle, promotes the growth of the uterine lining, and maintains vaginal health. Beyond reproduction, it plays a crucial role in bone health by promoting bone formation and inhibiting bone breakdown.

In the cardiovascular system, estrogen helps maintain the elasticity of blood vessels and promotes healthy cholesterol levels.

Estrogen's influence extends to the brain, where it affects mood, memory, and cognitive function. It modulates neurotransmitter systems, including serotonin and dopamine, which can impact your emotional well-being. Some research suggests that estrogen may even have neuroprotective effects, potentially reducing the risk of neurodegenerative diseases.

In the skin, estrogen promotes collagen production and helps maintain skin thickness and elasticity. It also influences fat distribution, contributing to the characteristic female body shape. Even the immune system feels the effects of estrogen, which can modulate immune responses and potentially impact autoimmune conditions.

As you transition through menopause, the decline in estrogen levels can lead to a host of symptoms and potential health risks. Hot flashes, night sweats, and mood swings are often the most noticeable short-term effects. Long-term consequences may include an increased risk of osteoporosis, cardiovascular disease, and cognitive decline.

Understanding this complex interplay of estrogen in your body underscores the importance of maintaining hormonal balance. While HRT can effectively address estrogen deficiency, your diet and lifestyle choices also play a crucial role in supporting your body's hormonal health.

Nourishing Your Hormones Through Diet

Your daily food choices significantly influence your hormonal balance. The Estrogen Matters Diet aims to support your body's hormonal health through strategic nutritional choices. By focusing on foods that naturally support estrogen production and balance, you can complement medical interventions like HRT or support your body's natural hormonal fluctuations.

Phytoestrogens, plant compounds that mimic estrogen in the body, play a central role in this dietary approach. Found in foods such as soybeans, flaxseeds, and certain fruits and vegetables, phytoestrogens can bind to estrogen receptors and exert mild estrogenic effects.

While not as potent as your body's natural estrogen or synthetic hormones used in HRT, these compounds may help alleviate some menopausal symptoms and offer potential health benefits.

Adding a variety of phytoestrogen-rich foods to your diet provides a gentle, natural way to support your hormonal balance. Soy products, such as tofu, tempeh, and edamame, are particularly rich sources. Flaxseeds and sesame seeds also offer significant amounts of these beneficial compounds. Fruits like apples, cherries, and dates, as well as vegetables such as carrots and fennel, can contribute to your phytoestrogen intake.

Beyond phytoestrogens, certain nutrients play crucial roles in hormone production and metabolism. Omega-3 fatty acids, found in fatty fish, walnuts, and chia seeds, support overall hormonal health and may help reduce inflammation. Vitamin D and calcium are essential for bone health, particularly important as estrogen levels decline. Magnesium, found in leafy greens, nuts, and whole grains, supports numerous bodily functions and may help alleviate some menopausal symptoms.

Cruciferous vegetables, such as broccoli, cauliflower, and Brussels sprouts, contain compounds that support healthy estrogen metabolism. These vegetables can help your body process and eliminate excess estrogen, promoting a balanced hormonal state.

Fiber-rich foods play a dual role in hormonal health. They help regulate blood sugar levels, which can impact hormone production, and also assist in the elimination of excess hormones through the digestive system. Include a variety of whole grains, legumes, fruits, and vegetables in your diet to ensure adequate fiber intake.

It's equally important to be mindful of foods that may negatively impact your hormonal balance. Excessive sugar and refined carbohydrates can lead to blood sugar spikes, potentially disrupting hormone levels. Processed foods often contain additives and preservatives that may interfere with hormonal function. Alcohol consumption can affect estrogen metabolism and potentially increase breast cancer risk, so moderation is key.

As you explore the recipes and meal plans in this cookbook, you'll find numerous options that incorporate these hormone-supporting foods. By nourishing your body with a balanced, nutrient-dense diet, you're providing the building blocks necessary for optimal hormonal function.

While diet plays a crucial role in hormonal health, it's just one aspect of overall well-being. Regular exercise, stress management, adequate sleep, and, when appropriate, medical interventions like HRT all contribute to your hormonal health. This culinary approach serves as a complementary strategy to a comprehensive health plan.

The following chapters will explore the specific dietary principles of the Estrogen Matters Diet, present a wide range of nutritious recipes, and offer practical tips for adding these hormone-supporting foods to your daily routine. By combining scientific knowledge with culinary creativity, you'll be equipped to make informed choices that support your hormonal health and overall well-being.

Chapter 1: Understanding Your Hormones

The human body is a complex network of systems working in concert to maintain health and vitality. At the heart of this intricate biological orchestra lies the endocrine system, a collection of glands that produce and secrete hormones. These chemical messengers play crucial roles in regulating numerous bodily functions, from metabolism and growth to reproduction and mood.

The Endocrine System: Your Body's Chemical Messaging Network

The endocrine system consists of several major glands distributed throughout your body. These include:

1. Hypothalamus: Located in the brain, this gland acts as a link between the nervous system and the endocrine system. It produces releasing and inhibiting hormones that control the pituitary gland.

2. Pituitary Gland: Often called the "master gland," the pituitary sits at the base of the brain and produces hormones that regulate other endocrine glands.

3. Thyroid Gland: Found in the neck, this gland produces thyroid hormones that regulate metabolism, growth, and development.

4. Parathyroid Glands: Four tiny glands located behind the thyroid that control calcium levels in the blood and bones.

5. Adrenal Glands: Situated atop the kidneys, these glands produce hormones involved in stress response, blood pressure regulation, and metabolism.

6. Pancreas: This organ produces insulin and glucagon, hormones that regulate blood sugar levels.

7. Ovaries (in women): These reproductive glands produce estrogen and progesterone, key hormones in the female reproductive cycle.

8. Testes (in men): The male reproductive glands produce testosterone, essential for male characteristics and reproductive function.

Each of these glands produces specific hormones that travel through the bloodstream to target cells or organs. When a hormone reaches its target, it binds to specific receptors, triggering a cascade of cellular responses. This system allows for precise control of various bodily functions, maintaining a state of balance known as homeostasis.

Key Hormones and Their Functions

Understanding the roles of specific hormones provides insight into how they influence your health and well-being. Here's an overview of some key hormones:

1. Estrogen:

Primarily produced by the ovaries in women, estrogen is crucial for female reproductive health. It regulates the menstrual cycle, supports pregnancy, and plays a role in bone health, cardiovascular function, and cognitive processes. During menopause, declining estrogen levels can lead to various symptoms and health concerns.

2. Progesterone:

Another female sex hormone, progesterone works in tandem with estrogen to regulate the menstrual cycle and support pregnancy. It helps prepare the uterus for implantation of a fertilized egg and maintains pregnancy.

3. Testosterone:

While often associated with men, testosterone is present in both sexes. In men, it's responsible for the development of male characteristics, sperm production, and muscle mass. In women, it contributes to libido and bone health.

4. Thyroid Hormones (T3 and T4):

Produced by the thyroid gland, these hormones regulate metabolism, body temperature, and energy levels. They influence nearly every organ system in the body.

5. Cortisol:

Often called the "stress hormone," cortisol is produced by the adrenal glands in response to stress. It helps regulate metabolism, immune function, and blood pressure.

6. Insulin:

Secreted by the pancreas, insulin allows cells to use glucose from the bloodstream for energy. It plays a crucial role in regulating blood sugar levels.

7. Growth Hormone:

Produced by the pituitary gland, growth hormone stimulates growth and cell reproduction. It's essential for childhood growth and continues to play a role in metabolism and muscle mass throughout adulthood.

8. Melatonin:

This hormone, produced by the pineal gland, regulates sleep-wake cycles. It's influenced by light exposure and helps maintain your body's circadian rhythm.

9. Oxytocin:

Often called the "love hormone," oxytocin is involved in social bonding, sexual reproduction, and childbirth. It's released during physical affection and plays a role in maternal behaviors.

10. Leptin and Ghrelin:

These hormones regulate hunger and satiety. Leptin, produced by fat cells, signals fullness, while ghrelin, produced in the stomach, stimulates appetite.

Hormonal Balance and Health

Your body's delicate equilibrium is maintained by the complex interaction of these hormones. Several health problems can develop when this equilibrium is upset. To illustrate:

- Thyroid imbalances can lead to weight changes, fatigue, and mood disturbances.
- Insulin resistance can result in type 2 diabetes.
- Imbalances in sex hormones can affect fertility, sexual function, and bone health.
- Cortisol imbalances can impact stress response, immune function, and metabolism.

Factors that can influence hormonal balance include:

1. Age: Hormone levels naturally change throughout life, with significant shifts occurring during puberty, pregnancy, and menopause.

2. Diet: Nutritional deficiencies or excesses can affect hormone production and function.

3. Stress: Chronic stress can disrupt the balance of several hormones, particularly cortisol.

4. Environmental factors: Exposure to certain chemicals, known as endocrine disruptors, can interfere with hormone function.

5. Medical conditions: Some health issues, such as polycystic ovary syndrome (PCOS) or thyroid disorders, directly affect hormone levels.

6. Medications: Certain medications, including hormonal birth control, can alter hormone levels.

Understanding these influences empowers you to make lifestyle choices that support hormonal health. A balanced diet, regular exercise, stress management, and adequate sleep all contribute to maintaining hormonal equilibrium.

The Endocrine System and Aging

As you age, your endocrine system undergoes changes that can affect overall health and well-being. The most significant hormonal shift for women occurs during menopause, typically in their late 40s or early 50s. During this transition, the ovaries gradually produce less estrogen and progesterone, leading to the cessation of menstrual periods and various symptoms such as hot flashes, mood changes, and vaginal dryness.

Men experience a more gradual decline in testosterone levels with age, a process sometimes referred to as andropause. This can result in decreased muscle mass, reduced bone density, and changes in sexual function.

Other age-related hormonal changes include:
- Decreased growth hormone production, which can affect body composition and energy levels.
- Reduced melatonin secretion, potentially leading to sleep disturbances.
- Changes in thyroid function, which can impact metabolism and energy.

These hormonal shifts contribute to many of the physical and emotional changes associated with aging. Understanding these processes allows for proactive steps to maintain health and vitality as you age.

Hormones and Women's Health

For women, hormones play a particularly crucial role throughout life, from puberty through menopause and beyond. The menstrual cycle involves a complex interplay of hormones, primarily estrogen and progesterone, that regulate ovulation and prepare the body for potential pregnancy.

During pregnancy, dramatic hormonal changes occur to support fetal development and prepare for childbirth. Estrogen and progesterone levels rise significantly, while other hormones like human chorionic gonadotropin (hCG) and relaxin play specific roles in maintaining pregnancy and preparing for delivery.

As women approach menopause, fluctuating hormone levels can lead to various symptoms. The perimenopause period, which can last several years, often involves irregular periods, hot flashes, mood changes, and sleep disturbances. After menopause, the decreased estrogen levels can increase the risk of certain health issues, including osteoporosis and cardiovascular disease.

Understanding these hormonal processes empowers women to make informed decisions about their health, including whether to consider hormone replacement therapy or other interventions to manage menopausal symptoms and reduce long-term health risks.

Hormones and Men's Health

While often less discussed, hormones play a significant role in men's health as well. Testosterone, the primary male sex hormone, influences numerous aspects of male physiology, including:

- Muscle mass and strength
- Bone density
- Fat distribution
- Red blood cell production
- Sperm production
- Sex drive

As men age, testosterone levels gradually decline, typically by about 1% per year after age 30. This natural decrease can contribute to various changes, including reduced muscle mass, increased body fat, decreased bone density, and changes in sexual function.

Other hormones, such as thyroid hormones and cortisol, also play crucial roles in men's health, affecting energy levels, metabolism, and stress response.

Recognizing the importance of hormonal health allows men to take proactive steps to maintain well-being as they age, potentially including lifestyle modifications or medical interventions when appropriate.

The Future of Hormone Research

Scientific understanding of the endocrine system continues to evolve, with ongoing research revealing new insights into hormone function and interactions. Emerging areas of study include:

- The role of hormones in mental health and cognitive function
- Interactions between hormones and the gut microbiome
- The impact of environmental endocrine disruptors on human health
- Personalized approaches to hormone therapy based on genetic profiles
- The potential of bioidentical hormones in treating hormonal imbalances

These advancements promise to enhance our ability to maintain hormonal balance and address hormone-related health issues more effectively in the future.

By grasping the fundamentals of the endocrine system and the functions of key hormones, you gain valuable insight into your body's intricate regulatory processes. This knowledge forms a foundation for understanding how diet, lifestyle, and medical interventions can support hormonal health throughout life's stages.

Menopause marks a significant transition in a woman's life, characterized by profound hormonal shifts that affect virtually every aspect of health and well-being. This natural biological process typically occurs between the ages of 45 and 55, signaling the end of reproductive years. The impact of menopause on hormonal balance is far-reaching, influencing not only reproductive function but also metabolism, bone health, cardiovascular function, and cognitive processes.

Hormonal Changes During Menopause

The primary hormonal change during menopause is the dramatic decline in estrogen production by the ovaries. This decrease occurs gradually over several years in a period known as perimenopause, eventually leading to the cessation of menstrual cycles. Alongside estrogen, levels of progesterone also fall significantly.

These hormonal shifts trigger a cascade of effects throughout the body:

1. Reproductive System:

The most immediate impact is on the reproductive system. As estrogen levels drop, the menstrual cycle becomes irregular before eventually stopping. The uterine lining thins, and vaginal tissue may become less elastic and more prone to dryness and irritation.

2. Vasomotor Symptoms:

Perhaps the most well-known menopausal symptoms, hot flashes and night sweats, result from the body's altered ability to regulate temperature due to hormonal changes. These vasomotor symptoms can significantly impact quality of life, disrupting sleep and daily activities.

3. Bone Health:

Estrogen is essential for regulating bone density, which brings us to our third point about bone health. Bone loss is accelerated during menopause, leading to an increased risk of osteoporosis and fractures, as its levels fall. This shift highlights the significance of postmenopausal women implementing steps to maintain bone health.

4. Cardiovascular System:

Estrogen exerts protective effects on the cardiovascular system. Its decrease during menopause is associated with an increased risk of heart disease and stroke. Changes in lipid profiles, with a tendency towards higher LDL (bad) cholesterol and lower HDL (good) cholesterol, contribute to this increased risk.

5. Metabolic Changes:

Hormonal shifts can affect metabolism and body composition. Many women experience weight gain, particularly around the abdomen, and changes in insulin sensitivity. These metabolic changes can increase the risk of type 2 diabetes.

6. Cognitive Function:

Some women report changes in memory and cognitive function during the menopausal transition. While the exact mechanisms are not fully understood, fluctuating hormone levels may influence neurotransmitter function and brain structure.

7. Mood and Mental Health:

Hormonal changes can impact mood, potentially contributing to increased risk of depression and anxiety during the menopausal transition. Sleep disturbances related to night sweats can exacerbate these effects.

8. Skin and Hair:

The decline in estrogen affects collagen production, leading to changes in skin elasticity and hydration. Some women may notice thinning hair or increased facial hair growth due to the altered balance of estrogen and androgens.

9. Urinary System:

Decreased estrogen can lead to thinning of the urethral lining, potentially causing urinary incontinence or increased susceptibility to urinary tract infections.

Adjusting to Changes in Hormones

The body's adaptation to these hormonal shifts varies among individuals. Some women experience minimal symptoms, while others face significant challenges. Several factors influence this adaptation process:

1. Genetics:

Family history can provide insights into how an individual might experience menopause. Genetic factors influence the timing of menopause and the severity of symptoms.

2. Lifestyle:

Diet, exercise habits, stress levels, and overall health status play crucial roles in how the body adapts to hormonal changes. A healthy lifestyle can mitigate some of the negative impacts of menopause.

3. Environmental Factors:

Exposure to endocrine-disrupting chemicals in the environment may influence hormonal balance and menopausal symptoms.

4. Pre-existing Health Conditions:

Women with certain health conditions may be more vulnerable to the effects of hormonal changes during menopause.

Strategies for Managing Hormonal Balance

While the hormonal changes of menopause are inevitable, various strategies can help manage their impact:

1. Dietary Approaches:

A balanced diet rich in phytoestrogens (plant compounds with estrogen-like effects) may help alleviate some menopausal symptoms. Foods like soy products, flaxseeds, and certain fruits and vegetables can be beneficial. Adequate calcium and vitamin D intake is crucial for bone health.

2. Regular Exercise:

Physical activity helps maintain a healthy weight, supports bone density, improves mood, and may reduce the frequency and severity of hot flashes.

3. Stress Management:

Techniques such as meditation, yoga, or deep breathing exercises can help manage stress, which can exacerbate menopausal symptoms.

4. Hormone Replacement Therapy (HRT):

For some women, HRT can effectively manage menopausal symptoms and potentially offer long-term health benefits. However, the decision to use HRT should be made in consultation with a healthcare provider, considering individual health history and risk factors.

5. Non-Hormonal Medications:

Various medications can target specific menopausal symptoms, such as antidepressants for mood changes or hot flashes, or medications to prevent bone loss.

6. Complementary Therapies:

Some women find relief from menopausal symptoms through acupuncture, herbal remedies, or other alternative therapies. It's important to discuss these options with a healthcare provider to ensure safety and efficacy.

7. Lifestyle Modifications:

Simple changes like dressing in layers, avoiding trigger foods for hot flashes, and maintaining a cool sleeping environment can help manage symptoms.

Long-Term Health Considerations

The hormonal changes of menopause have implications for long-term health that extend beyond the immediate symptoms:

1. Osteoporosis Prevention:

Strategies to maintain bone density become increasingly important. This may include calcium and vitamin D supplementation, weight-bearing exercises, and in some cases, medications to prevent bone loss.

2. Cardiovascular Health:

Postmenopausal women should pay particular attention to heart health through diet, exercise, and regular check-ups to monitor blood pressure, cholesterol levels, and other cardiovascular risk factors.

3. Cancer Risk:

While the risk of certain cancers, such as ovarian cancer, decreases after menopause, the risk of breast cancer may increase. Regular screenings and awareness of changes in breast tissue are important.

4. Sexual Health:

Addressing changes in sexual function and maintaining intimacy may require open communication with partners and healthcare providers. Lubricants, vaginal moisturizers, or local estrogen treatments can help manage vaginal dryness and discomfort.

5. Cognitive Health:

Engaging in mentally stimulating activities, maintaining social connections, and staying physically active may help support cognitive function as hormone levels change.

Chapter 2: The Estrogen Matters Diet Principles

The Estrogen Matters Diet Principles are founded on the understanding that nutrition plays a crucial role in supporting hormonal balance, particularly in relation to estrogen. This approach focuses on incorporating foods and nutrients that support estrogen production and balance, while limiting those that may disrupt hormonal equilibrium. Now, let's go into these fundamentals.

Foods that Support Estrogen Production and Balance

1. Phytoestrogen-Rich Foods:

Phytoestrogens are plant compounds that can mimic estrogen in the body. While not as potent as endogenous estrogen, they can help alleviate some symptoms of estrogen deficiency. Key sources include:

a) Soy products: Tofu, tempeh, edamame, and soy milk contain isoflavones, a type of phytoestrogen.
- Flaxseeds: Rich in lignans, another type of phytoestrogen.
- Sesame seeds: Also contain lignans and other beneficial compounds.
- Legumes: Chickpeas, lentils, and other beans offer phytoestrogens and fiber.
- Fruits: Berries, peaches, and dried fruits like dates and prunes contain varying levels of phytoestrogens.
b) Vegetables: Cruciferous vegetables like broccoli, cauliflower, and Brussels sprouts contain indole-3-carbinol, which supports healthy estrogen metabolism.

2. Fiber-Rich Foods:

Dietary fiber plays a crucial role in hormonal balance by helping to regulate estrogen levels. It can bind to excess estrogen in the digestive tract, facilitating its elimination from the body. Good sources include:
- Whole grains: Oats, quinoa, brown rice, and whole wheat products.
- Vegetables: Leafy greens, carrots, beets, and artichokes.
- Fruits: Apples, pears, and berries.
- Legumes: All types of beans, lentils, and peas.

3. Omega-3 Fatty Acids:

These essential fats support overall hormonal health and can help reduce inflammation. Sources include:

- Fatty fish: Salmon, mackerel, sardines, and trout.
- Walnuts and chia seeds.
- Flaxseeds and flaxseed oil.
- Algae-based supplements for vegetarians and vegans.

4. Healthy Fats:

Adequate fat intake is crucial for hormone production. Focus on:

- Avocados
- Olive oil
- Nuts and seeds
- Coconut oil (in moderation)

5. Fermented Foods:

These support gut health, which is closely linked to hormonal balance. Include:

- Yogurt and kefir
- Sauerkraut
- Kimchi
- Kombucha

Nutrients Essential for Hormonal Health

1. B Vitamins:

B vitamins play various roles in hormone production and metabolism. Key sources include:

- B6: Found in poultry, fish, potatoes, and non-citrus fruits.
- B9 (Folate): Abundant in leafy greens, legumes, and fortified grains.
- B12: Primarily found in animal products; vegans may need supplementation.

2. Vitamin D:

This vitamin acts more like a hormone in the body and supports overall endocrine function. Sources include:

- Sunlight exposure
- Fatty fish
- Egg yolks
- Fortified foods
- Supplements (often necessary, especially in northern latitudes)

3. Magnesium:

Essential for over 300 enzymatic reactions in the body, including hormone production. Good sources are:

- Dark leafy greens
- Nuts and seeds
- Whole grains
- Dark chocolate

4. Zinc:

Crucial for reproductive health and hormone production. Find it in:

- Oysters
- Beef
- Pumpkin seeds
- Lentils

5. Selenium:

Supports thyroid function, which is closely tied to overall hormonal balance. Sources include:

- Brazil nuts
- Fish
- Poultry
- Whole grains

6. Iodine:

Essential for thyroid hormone production. Sources include:

- Seaweed
- Iodized salt
- Fish
- Dairy products

7. Vitamin E:

An antioxidant that supports overall cellular health, including hormone-producing cells. Find it in:

- Sunflower seeds
- Almonds
- Avocados
- Spinach

Foods to Avoid or Limit

1. Processed Foods:

Many processed foods contain additives and preservatives that may disrupt hormonal balance. These include:

- Packaged snacks
- Processed meats
- Many fast food items
- Foods with artificial colors or flavors

2. Excess Sugar:

High sugar intake can lead to insulin resistance and hormonal imbalances. Limit:

- Sugary drinks
- Candies and sweets
- Baked goods
- Hidden sugars in sauces and dressings

3. Alcohol:

Excessive alcohol consumption can disrupt hormone production and metabolism. If consumed, do so in moderation.

4. Caffeine:

While moderate caffeine intake is generally fine for most people, excessive consumption can impact hormone levels and sleep quality.

These artificial fats can promote inflammation and disrupt hormone function. Avoid:
- Fried foods
- Many baked goods
- Some margarines
- Foods containing partially hydrogenated oils

While fish is generally healthy, some types high in mercury can negatively impact hormonal health. Limit intake of:
- Shark
- Swordfish
- King mackerel
- Tilefish

Certain chemicals can mimic or interfere with hormone function. While not foods themselves, be mindful of:
- BPA in some plastic containers and can linings
- Pesticides on non-organic produce
- Phthalates in some food packaging

Implementing the Estrogen Matters Diet Principles

Adopting these dietary principles doesn't mean a complete overhaul of your eating habits. Instead, focus on gradually incorporating more hormone-supportive foods while reducing those that may disrupt balance. Here are some practical tips:

1. Build your meals around plant-based proteins, whole grains, and plenty of vegetables.

2. Include a serving of phytoestrogen-rich foods daily, such as a handful of flaxseeds in your morning smoothie or a tofu stir-fry for dinner.

3. Aim for at least 25-30 grams of fiber per day through a variety of fruits, vegetables, whole grains, and legumes.

4. Incorporate fatty fish into your diet 2-3 times per week, or consider a high-quality omega-3 supplement.

5. Snack on nuts and seeds for healthy fats and important minerals.

6. Choose organic produce when possible, especially for the "Dirty Dozen" – fruits and vegetables most likely to have pesticide residues.

7. Stay hydrated with water, herbal teas, and unsweetened beverages.

8. Experiment with new recipes that incorporate a variety of hormone-supportive foods.

9. Practice mindful eating, paying attention to hunger and fullness cues.

10. Remember that no single food is a magic bullet – consistency and variety are key.

Personalization and Consultation

While these principles provide a solid foundation for hormone-supportive nutrition, individual needs may vary. Factors such as age, overall health status, specific hormonal imbalances, and personal food preferences should be considered. It's advisable to consult with a healthcare provider or registered dietitian who can help tailor these guidelines to your specific needs.

For women undergoing menopause or experiencing significant hormonal changes, additional dietary modifications or supplements may be recommended. Similarly, those with conditions such as thyroid disorders, PCOS, or endometriosis may benefit from more targeted nutritional strategies.

Chapter 3: Meal Planning to Achieve Hormonal Balance

Meal planning is a powerful tool for supporting hormonal balance. By creating well-structured, nutrient-dense meals, you can provide your body with the essential building blocks it needs to maintain optimal hormone function. This chapter will guide you through the process of creating balanced meals, managing portion sizes, and implementing effective meal prep strategies.

Creating Balanced Meals

The foundation of hormone-supportive meal planning lies in creating balanced meals that incorporate a variety of nutrients. Here's how to structure your meals for optimal hormonal health:

1. Protein:

Include a source of high-quality protein in each meal. Protein provides essential amino acids necessary for hormone production and helps stabilize blood sugar levels. Try to get 20-30 grams of protein with each intake.

Options include:

- Lean meats (chicken, turkey, lean beef)
- Fish (salmon, tuna, sardines)
- Eggs
- Legumes (lentils, chickpeas, black beans)
- Tofu or tempeh
- Greek yogurt

2. Complex Carbohydrates:

Choose fiber-rich, complex carbohydrates that provide sustained energy and support gut health. These carbs help regulate insulin levels, which is crucial for hormonal balance. Good choices include:

- Whole grains (quinoa, brown rice, oats)
- Sweet potatoes
- Butternut squash
- Berries
- Apples
- Legumes

3. Healthy Fats:

Incorporate sources of healthy fats, which are essential for hormone production and absorption of fat-soluble vitamins.
Include:

- Avocado
- Nuts and seeds (almonds, walnuts, chia seeds)
- Olive oil
- Fatty fish
- Coconut (in moderation)

4. Vegetables:

Fill at least half your plate with a variety of colorful vegetables. These provide fiber, vitamins, minerals, and antioxidants that support overall health and hormone function.
Focus on:

- Leafy greens (spinach, kale, collards)
- Cruciferous vegetables (broccoli, cauliflower, Brussels sprouts)
- Colorful bell peppers
- Carrots
- Beets

5. Hormone-Supportive Foods:

Incorporate foods known to support hormonal balance, such as those rich in phytoestrogens or specific nutrients.
Examples include:

- Flaxseeds
- Soy products (if well-tolerated)
- Fermented foods (sauerkraut, kimchi)
- Seaweed (for iodine)
- Brazil nuts (for selenium)

Meal Structure Examples:

Breakfast:

- Greek yogurt topped with berries, flaxseeds, and a handful of almonds
- Vegetable omelet with whole grain toast and avocado

Lunch:
- Grilled chicken salad with mixed greens, quinoa, and olive oil dressing
- Lentil soup with a side of roasted vegetables and pumpkin seeds

Dinner:
- Baked salmon with roasted sweet potato and steamed broccoli
- Tofu and vegetable stir-fry over brown rice

Portion Control

Proper portion control is crucial for maintaining a healthy weight and supporting hormonal balance. Here are strategies to help you manage portion sizes:

1. Use Smaller Plates:

Opt for 9-inch plates instead of larger ones to naturally reduce portion sizes.

2. Follow the Plate Method:
- Fill half your plate with non-starchy vegetables
- One-quarter with lean protein
- One-quarter with complex carbohydrates
- Add a small amount of healthy fat

3. Use Your Hand as a Guide:
- Protein: Palm-sized portion
- Carbohydrates: Cupped hand
- Vegetables: Two fists
- Fats: Thumb-sized portion

4. Be Mindful of Calorie-Dense Foods:

While nuts, seeds, and oils are healthy, they're also calorie-dense. Measure these portions carefully.

5. Listen to Your Body:

Eat slowly and stop when you feel satisfied, not overly full.

6. Stay Hydrated:

Sometimes thirst can be mistaken for hunger. Drink water throughout the day.

7. Limit Liquid Calories:

Be aware of calories from beverages, including smoothies and juices.

Meal Prep Tips and Tricks

Effective meal prep can make it easier to stick to your hormone-supportive eating plan.
Here are some strategies to streamline your meal preparation:

1. Plan Your Menu:
- Set aside time each week to plan your meals
- Create a grocery list based on your meal plan
- Consider theme nights (e.g., Meatless Monday, Taco Tuesday) for easier planning

2. Batch Cook Staples:
- Prepare large batches of grains, legumes, and roasted vegetables
- Cook extra protein to use in multiple meals
- Make big batches of soups or stews to portion and freeze

3. Prep Ingredients in Advance:
- Wash and chop vegetables for the week
- Portion out snacks into grab-and-go containers
- Marinate proteins for easy cooking later

4. Purchase High-Quality Storage Containers:
- Use glass containers for better food preservation and reheating
- Label containers with contents and date prepared

5. Utilize Your Freezer:
- Freeze individual portions of soups, stews, and casseroles
- Freeze overripe fruits for smoothies
- Store nuts and seeds in the freezer to extend shelf life

6. Create a Smoothie Station:
- Pre-portion smoothie ingredients into freezer bags
- Include a mix of fruits, vegetables, and add-ins like flaxseeds

7. Make Use of Time-Saving Appliances:

- Use a slow cooker or Instant Pot for hands-off cooking
- Consider a food processor for quick chopping and sauce-making

8. Prepare Grab-and-Go Options:

- Hard-boiled eggs
- Cut vegetables with hummus
- Homemade trail mix with nuts and seeds

9. Cook Once, Eat Twice:

- Plan meals that can be repurposed (e.g., grilled chicken for salad one day, tacos the next)
- Transform leftovers into new meals (e.g., leftover roasted vegetables in a frittata)

10. Keep a Well-Stocked Pantry:

- Maintain a supply of canned beans, whole grains, and nuts
- Stock frozen vegetables and fruits for quick meal additions

11. Practice Safe Food Handling:

- Cool foods properly before refrigerating
- Use the "first in, first out" method to rotate your ingredients
- Follow proper food safety guidelines for storage times

Implementing Your Meal Plan

As you begin implementing your hormone-supportive meal plan, keep these points in mind:

1. Start Gradually:

If this way of eating is new to you, start by incorporating one or two balanced meals per day and gradually increase.

2. Be Flexible:

Life happens, and your meal plan should be adaptable. Have backup options for busy days.

3. Listen to Your Body:
 Take note of how certain foods make you feel and modify your plan as necessary.

4. Maintain Hydration:
 Hormone activity depends on getting enough water in the body. Try to have eight glasses of water or more each day.

5. Consider Timing:
Some people find that eating larger meals earlier in the day and lighter meals in the evening supports better sleep and hormone balance.

6. Don't Forget Snacks:
Plan for nutritious snacks to maintain stable blood sugar levels throughout the day.

7. Celebrate Progress:
Acknowledge the positive changes you're making and be patient with yourself as you develop new habits.

Chapter 4: Breakfast recipes

Overnight Chia Seed Pudding

Prep Time: 10 minutes
Cooking Time: (Refrigerate overnight)
Serving Size: 2

Ingredients:

- 1/2 cup chia seeds
- 2 cups almond milk (or any milk of choice)
- 1-2 tablespoons honey or maple syrup
- 1 teaspoon vanilla extract
- Fresh berries, nuts, or granola for topping

Instructions:

1. In a mixing bowl, combine chia seeds, almond milk, honey (or maple syrup), and vanilla extract. Stir well.

2. Let the mixture sit for about 10 minutes, then stir again to break up any clumps.

3. Cover the bowl and refrigerate overnight.

4. In the morning, give the pudding a good stir. If it's too thick, add a little more milk until you reach your desired consistency.

5. Serve topped with fresh berries, nuts, or granola.

Nutritional Value (per serving): Calories 200, Fat 12g, Carbohydrates 18g, Fiber 10g, Protein 6g, Sugars 8g, Sodium 150mg

Spinach and Feta Egg Muffins

Prep Time: 10 minutes
Cooking Time: 20 minutes
Serving Size: 4 (makes 12 muffins)

Ingredients:
- 6 large eggs
- 1 cup fresh spinach, chopped
- 1/2 cup feta cheese, crumbled
- 1/4 cup milk
- 1/2 teaspoon salt
- 1/4 teaspoon black pepper
- 1/4 teaspoon garlic powder

Instructions:
1. Preheat your oven to 350°F (175°C) and grease a 12-cup muffin tin.
2. In a large mixing bowl, whisk together eggs and milk.
3. Stir in chopped spinach, feta cheese, salt, pepper, and garlic powder.
4. Pour the egg mixture evenly into the muffin tin cups.
5. Bake for 20 minutes or until the muffins are set and lightly golden.
6. Let cool slightly before removing from the tin. Serve warm or store in the refrigerator for up to 3 days.

Nutritional Value (per serving):
Calories 120, Fat 8g, Carbohydrates 2g, Fiber 1g, Protein 10g, Sugars 1g, Sodium 300mg

Avocado Toast with Smoked Salmon

Prep Time: 10 minutes
Cooking Time: 0
Serving Size: 1

Ingredients:
- 1 slice whole grain bread
- 1/2 ripe avocado
- 2 slices smoked salmon
- 1 teaspoon lemon juice
- Salt and pepper to taste
- Optional: capers, red onion slices, or fresh dill for garnish

Instructions:
1. Toast the slice of whole grain bread to your liking.
2. In a small bowl, mash the avocado with lemon juice, salt, and pepper.
3. Spread the mashed avocado on the toasted bread.
4. Top with smoked salmon slices.
5. Add optional garnishes like capers, red onion slices, or fresh dill if desired.

Nutritional Value (per serving):

Calories 300, Fat 20g, Carbohydrates 20g, Fiber 8g, Protein 12g, Sugars 2g, Sodium 600mg

Greek Yogurt Parfait with Berries and Flaxseeds

Prep Time: 5 minutes
Cooking Time: 0
Serving Size: 1

Ingredients:
- 1 cup Greek yogurt
- 1/2 cup mixed berries (blueberries, strawberries, raspberries)
- 1 tablespoon honey or maple syrup
- 1 tablespoon ground flaxseeds
- Optional: granola for topping

Instructions:
1. In a bowl or jar, layer Greek yogurt and mixed berries.
2. Drizzle with honey or maple syrup.
3. Sprinkle ground flaxseeds on top.
4. Add granola if using. Serve immediately.

Nutritional Value (per serving):
 Calories 250, Fat 8g, Carbohydrates 30g, Fiber 6g, Protein 15g, Sugars 20g, Sodium 70mg

Whole Grain Breakfast Smoothie Bowl

Prep Time: 10 minutes
Cooking Time: 0
Serving Size: 1

Ingredients:

- 1/2 cup rolled oats
- 1 cup unsweetened almond milk (or any milk of choice)
- 1 banana, sliced
- 1/2 cup mixed berries (frozen or fresh)
- 1 tablespoon almond butter
- 1 tablespoon chia seeds
- Optional: granola, fresh fruit, nuts for topping

Instructions:

1. In a blender, combine rolled oats, almond milk, banana, mixed berries, almond butter, and chia seeds. Blend until smooth.
2. Pour the smoothie into a bowl.
3. Top with granola, fresh fruit, and nuts if desired. Serve immediately.

Nutritional Value (per serving):

 Calories 350, Fat 12g, Carbohydrates 55g, Fiber 12g, Protein 10g, Sugars 20g, Sodium 150mg

Quinoa Vegetable Frittata

Prep Time: 15 minutes
Cooking Time: 25 minutes
Serving Size: 4

Ingredients:
- 1/2 cup quinoa, rinsed
- 1 cup water
- 1 tablespoon olive oil
- 1 small onion, diced
- 1 bell pepper, diced
- 1 zucchini, diced
- 1 cup baby spinach
- 6 large eggs
- 1/4 cup milk
- 1/2 teaspoon salt
- 1/4 teaspoon black pepper
- 1/4 cup feta cheese, crumbled

Instructions:
1. Preheat your oven to 375°F (190°C).
2. In a small pot, combine quinoa and water. Bring to a boil, then reduce heat and simmer for 15 minutes, or until water is absorbed. Set aside.
3. In an oven-safe skillet, heat olive oil over medium heat. Add onion and bell pepper, and sauté until softened.
4. Add zucchini and spinach, cooking until spinach wilts.
5. In a bowl, whisk together eggs, milk, salt, and pepper.
6. Stir in cooked quinoa and vegetables. Pour the mixture into the skillet.
7. Sprinkle feta cheese on top and transfer the skillet to the oven.
8. Bake for 20-25 minutes, or until the frittata is set and golden on top.
9. Let cool slightly before slicing and serving.

Nutritional Value (per serving):
Calories 250, Fat 14g, Carbohydrates 18g, Fiber 3g, Protein 12g, Sugars 4g, Sodium 450mg

Buckwheat Pancakes with Blueberry Compote

Prep Time: 10 minutes
Cooking Time: 20 minutes
Serving Size: 4

Ingredients:
Pancakes:
 - 1 cup buckwheat flour
 - 1/2 teaspoon baking soda
 - 1/4 teaspoon salt
 - 1 cup buttermilk
 - 1 large egg
 - 2 tablespoons melted butter
Blueberry Compote:
 - 1 cup fresh or frozen blueberries
 - 2 tablespoons maple syrup
 - 1 teaspoon lemon juice

Instructions:
1. Pancakes:
   1. In a large bowl, whisk together buckwheat flour, baking soda, and salt.
   2. In another bowl, mix buttermilk, egg, and melted butter.
   3. Combine wet and dry ingredients, stirring until just combined.
   4. Heat a non-stick skillet over medium heat and grease lightly.
   5. Pour 1/4 cup batter for each pancake and cook until bubbles form on the surface, then flip and cook until golden brown.
2. Blueberry Compote:
   1. In a small saucepan, combine blueberries, maple syrup, and lemon juice.
   2. Cook over medium heat until blueberries break down and the mixture thickens.
3. Serve pancakes with warm blueberry compote.

Nutritional Value (per serving):
Calories 250, Fat 9g, Carbohydrates 38g, Fiber 4g, Protein 6g, Sugars 10g, Sodium 400mg

Shakshuka with Whole Grain Pita

Prep Time: 10 minutes
Cooking Time: 20 minutes
Serving Size: 4

Ingredients:
- 1 tablespoon olive oil
- 1 onion, diced
- 1 red bell pepper, diced
- 3 cloves garlic, minced
- 1 teaspoon ground cumin
- 1 teaspoon paprika
- 1/4 teaspoon cayenne pepper
- 1 can (28 oz) diced tomatoes
- 1/4 cup tomato sauce
- 4 large eggs
- Salt and pepper to taste
- Fresh cilantro or parsley, chopped (for garnish)
- Whole grain pita bread

Instructions:
1. In a large skillet, heat olive oil over medium heat.
2. Add onion and bell pepper, sauté until softened.
3. Stir in garlic, cumin, paprika, and cayenne pepper, cooking until fragrant.
4. Add diced tomatoes and tomato sauce, simmer for 10 minutes until slightly thickened.
5. Make four small wells in the sauce and crack an egg into each well.
6. Cover the skillet and cook until the eggs are set to your liking.
7. Season with salt and pepper, garnish with fresh cilantro or parsley.
8. Serve with warm whole grain pita bread.

Nutritional Value (per serving):
Calories 200, Fat 10g, Carbohydrates 20g, Fiber 5g, Protein 10g, Sugars 8g, Sodium 500mg

Sweet Potato and Black Bean Breakfast Burrito

Prep Time: 15 minutes
Cooking Time: 20 minutes
Serving Size: 4

Ingredients:
- 1 large sweet potato, peeled and diced
- 1 tablespoon olive oil
- 1 small onion, diced
- 1 bell pepper, diced
- 1 can (15 oz) black beans, rinsed and drained
- 1 teaspoon cumin
- 1/2 teaspoon chili powder
- Salt and pepper to taste
- 4 large whole grain tortillas
- 1/2 cup shredded cheddar cheese
- Salsa and avocado slices for serving

Instructions:
1. In a skillet, heat olive oil over medium heat. Add sweet potato and cook until tender.
2. Add onion and bell pepper, sauté until softened.
3. Stir in black beans, cumin, chili powder, salt, and pepper. Cook until heated through.
4. Warm the tortillas and divide the sweet potato mixture among them.
5. Sprinkle with shredded cheese, then roll up into burritos.
6. Serve with salsa and avocado slices.

Nutritional Value (per serving):
Calories 350, Fat 12g, Carbohydrates 50g, Fiber 10g, Protein 12g, Sugars 5g, Sodium 600mg

Smoked Tofu and Vegetable Scramble

Prep Time: 10 minutes
Cooking Time: 15 minutes
Serving Size: 4

Ingredients:
- 1 tablespoon olive oil
- 1 block smoked tofu, crumbled
- 1 small onion, diced
- 1 bell pepper, diced
- 1 zucchini, diced
- 1 cup cherry tomatoes, halved
- 1/2 teaspoon turmeric
- Salt and pepper to taste
- Fresh basil or parsley, chopped (for garnish)

Instructions:
1. In a large skillet, heat olive oil over medium heat.
2. Add onion and bell pepper, sauté until softened.
3. Stir in zucchini and cherry tomatoes, cooking until tender.
4. Add crumbled smoked tofu and turmeric, mixing well.
5. Cook until the tofu is heated through. Season with salt and pepper.
6. Garnish with fresh basil or parsley and serve warm.

Nutritional Value (per serving):
Calories 200, Fat 10g, Carbohydrates 15g, Fiber 5g, Protein 15g, Sugars 5g, Sodium 400mg

Baked Oatmeal Cups with Apples and Walnuts

Prep Time: 15 minutes
Cooking Time: 25 minutes
Serving Size: 12 cups

Ingredients:
- 2 cups rolled oats
- 1 teaspoon baking powder
- 1/2 teaspoon cinnamon
- 1/4 teaspoon salt
- 1 1/2 cups milk (any type)
- 2 large eggs
- 1/4 cup maple syrup
- 1 teaspoon vanilla extract
- 1 apple, peeled, cored, and diced
- 1/2 cup walnuts, chopped

Instructions:
1. Preheat your oven to 350°F (175°C) and grease a 12-cup muffin tin.
2. In a large bowl, combine rolled oats, baking powder, cinnamon, and salt.
3. In another bowl, whisk together milk, eggs, maple syrup, and vanilla extract.
4. Pour the wet ingredients into the dry ingredients and mix well.
5. Fold in diced apples and chopped walnuts.
6. Divide the mixture evenly among the muffin cups.
7. Bake for 20-25 minutes, or until the oatmeal cups are set and golden brown.
8. Let cool completely before storing in the refrigerator for up to a week or in the freezer for up to 3 months.

Nutritional Value (per cup):
 Calories 150, Fat 7g, Carbohydrates 20g, Fiber 3g, Protein 4g, Sugars 8g, Sodium 100mg

Veggie-Packed Breakfast Casserole

Prep Time: 20 minutes
Cooking Time: 45 minutes
Serving Size: 8

Ingredients:
- 1 tablespoon olive oil
- 1 onion, diced
- 1 bell pepper, diced
- 1 zucchini, diced
- 1 cup spinach, chopped
- 8 large eggs
- 1 cup milk (any type)
- 1/2 teaspoon salt
- 1/4 teaspoon black pepper
- 1/4 teaspoon garlic powder
- 1 cup shredded cheddar cheese

Instructions:
1. Preheat your oven to 375°F (190°C) and grease a 9x13-inch baking dish.
2. In a large skillet, heat olive oil over medium heat. Add onion and bell pepper, sauté until softened.
3. Add zucchini and spinach, cooking until the spinach wilts.
4. In a large bowl, whisk together eggs, milk, salt, pepper, and garlic powder.
5. Stir in the cooked vegetables and shredded cheese.
6. Pour the mixture into the prepared baking dish.
7. Bake for 35-45 minutes, or until the casserole is set and golden brown on top.
8. Let cool completely before slicing and storing in the refrigerator for up to 5 days or in the freezer for up to 3 months.

Nutritional Value (per serving):
Calories 200, Fat 12g, Carbohydrates 8g, Fiber 2g, Protein 15g, Sugars 4g, Sodium 350mg

Protein-Rich Breakfast Cookies

Prep Time: 10 minutes
Cooking Time: 15 minutes
Serving Size: 12 cookies

Ingredients:
- 1 cup rolled oats
- 1/2 cup almond flour
- 1/4 cup protein powder (optional)
- 1 teaspoon baking powder
- 1/2 teaspoon cinnamon
- 1/4 teaspoon salt
- 1/4 cup almond butter
- 1/4 cup maple syrup
- 1 large egg
- 1 teaspoon vanilla extract
- 1/2 cup raisins or chocolate chips

Instructions:
1. Preheat your oven to 350°F (175°C) and line a baking sheet with parchment paper.
2. In a large bowl, combine rolled oats, almond flour, protein powder, baking powder, cinnamon, and salt.
3. In another bowl, mix almond butter, maple syrup, egg, and vanilla extract.
4. Pour the wet ingredients into the dry ingredients and mix well.
5. Fold in raisins or chocolate chips.
6. Scoop 2 tablespoons of dough for each cookie and place on the baking sheet, flattening slightly.
7. Bake for 12-15 minutes, or until the cookies are golden brown.
8. Let cool completely before storing in an airtight container for up to a week.

Nutritional Value (per cookie):
 Calories 150, Fat 7g, Carbohydrates 18g, Fiber 3g, Protein 6g, Sugars 8g, Sodium 100mg

Mason Jar Layered Greek Yogurt Parfaits

Prep Time: 10 minutes
Cooking Time: 0
Serving Size: 4

Ingredients:
- 2 cups Greek yogurt
- 1 cup granola
- 1 cup mixed berries (blueberries, strawberries, raspberries)
- 2 tablespoons honey or maple syrup
- 4 mason jars

Instructions:
1. In each mason jar, start with a layer of Greek yogurt (about 1/2 cup).
2. Add a layer of mixed berries (about 1/4 cup).
3. Drizzle with honey or maple syrup (about 1/2 tablespoon).
4. Add a layer of granola (about 1/4 cup).
5. Repeat the layers if desired.
6. Seal the jars with lids and refrigerate for up to 5 days.

Nutritional Value (per serving):
 Calories 250, Fat 9g, Carbohydrates 30g, Fiber 5g, Protein 15g, Sugars 20g, Sodium 100mg

Freezer-Friendly Breakfast Burritos

Prep Time: 20 minutes
Cooking Time: 10 minutes
Serving Size: 8

Ingredients:
- 1 tablespoon olive oil
- 1 onion, diced
- 1 bell pepper, diced
- 1 cup cooked black beans
- 8 large eggs
- 1/4 cup milk (any type)
- Salt and pepper to taste
- 8 large whole grain tortillas
- 1 cup shredded cheddar cheese
- Salsa for serving

Instructions:
1. In a large skillet, heat olive oil over medium heat. Add onion and bell pepper, sauté until softened.
2. Stir in cooked black beans and cook until heated through.
3. In a bowl, whisk together eggs, milk, salt, and pepper.
4. Pour the egg mixture into the skillet and cook, stirring occasionally, until scrambled and set.
5. Warm the tortillas and divide the egg mixture among them.
6. Sprinkle with shredded cheese, then roll up into burritos.
7. Wrap each burrito in foil and place in a freezer-safe bag. Freeze for up to 3 months.
8. To reheat, remove foil and microwave on high for 2-3 minutes, or until heated through.

Nutritional Value (per burrito):
Calories 300, Fat 15g, Carbohydrates 30g, Fiber 5g, Protein 15g, Sugars 4g, Sodium 600mg

Chapter 5: Lunch Recipes
Lentil and Roasted Vegetable Grain Bowl

Prep Time: 15 minutes
Cooking Time: 30 minutes
Serving Size: 4

Ingredients:
- 1 cup green or brown lentils
- 2 cups vegetable broth
- 1 sweet potato, peeled and diced
- 1 red bell pepper, diced
- 1 zucchini, diced
- 2 tablespoons olive oil
- Salt and pepper to taste
- 1 cup cooked quinoa or farro
- 2 cups baby spinach
- 1 avocado, sliced
- 1/4 cup feta cheese, crumbled (optional)
- Balsamic vinaigrette for dressing

Instructions:
1. Preheat your oven to 400°F (200°C).
2. In a pot, combine lentils and vegetable broth. Bring to a boil, then reduce heat and simmer for 20-25 minutes, or until lentils are tender. Drain and set aside.
3. On a baking sheet, toss sweet potato, bell pepper, and zucchini with olive oil, salt, and pepper. Roast for 20-25 minutes, or until vegetables are tender and slightly browned.
4. In a large bowl, combine cooked lentils, roasted vegetables, cooked quinoa (or farro), and baby spinach.
5. Divide the mixture into bowls and top with avocado slices and feta cheese, if using.
6. Drizzle with balsamic vinaigrette before serving.

Nutritional Value (per serving):
Calories 350, Fat 14g, Carbohydrates 45g, Fiber 12g, Protein 12g, Sugars 8g, Sodium 400mg

Chickpea Salad Stuffed Pita Pockets

Prep Time: 15 minutes
Cooking Time: 0
Serving Size: 4

Ingredients:
- 1 can (15 oz) chickpeas, rinsed and drained
- 1/2 cup Greek yogurt
- 1 tablespoon lemon juice
- 1 teaspoon Dijon mustard
- 1 celery stalk, finely chopped
- 1 small red onion, finely chopped
- 1 small cucumber, diced
- 1/4 cup fresh parsley, chopped
- Salt and pepper to taste
- 4 whole grain pita pockets
- Mixed greens or lettuce leaves

Instructions:
1. In a large bowl, mash the chickpeas with a fork until slightly chunky.
2. Add Greek yogurt, lemon juice, Dijon mustard, celery, red onion, cucumber, parsley, salt, and pepper. Mix well to combine.
3. Cut pita pockets in half and gently open them.
4. Stuff each pita pocket with chickpea salad and mixed greens or lettuce leaves.
5. Serve immediately or wrap and refrigerate for up to 2 days.

Nutritional Value (per serving):
Calories 300, Fat 8g, Carbohydrates 45g, Fiber 10g, Protein 12g, Sugars 4g, Sodium 450mg

Sesame Ginger Tofu Lettuce Wraps

Prep Time: 15 minutes
Cooking Time: 10 minutes
Serving Size: 4

Ingredients:
- 1 block (14 oz) firm tofu, drained and crumbled
- 1 tablespoon sesame oil
- 2 cloves garlic, minced
- 1 tablespoon fresh ginger, grated
- 2 tablespoons soy sauce
- 1 tablespoon hoisin sauce
- 1 tablespoon rice vinegar
- 1 cup shredded carrots
- 1 cup shredded red cabbage
- 1/4 cup green onions, chopped
- 8 large lettuce leaves (butter lettuce or romaine works well)
- Sesame seeds for garnish

Instructions:
1. In a large skillet, heat sesame oil over medium-high heat. Add crumbled tofu and cook until browned, about 5 minutes.
2. Add garlic and ginger, cooking until fragrant, about 1 minute.
3. Stir in soy sauce, hoisin sauce, and rice vinegar. Cook for another 2-3 minutes, until the sauce is absorbed.
4. Remove from heat and mix in shredded carrots, red cabbage, and green onions.
5. Spoon the tofu mixture into lettuce leaves.
6. Garnish with sesame seeds and serve.

Nutritional Value (per serving):
Calories 250, Fat 12g, Carbohydrates 18g, Fiber 5g, Protein 16g, Sugars 6g, Sodium 500mg

Mediterranean Quinoa Salad with Grilled Chicken

Prep Time: 15 minutes
Cooking Time: 15 minutes
Serving Size: 4

Ingredients:
- 1 cup quinoa, rinsed
- 2 cups water
- 2 cups cooked, chopped grilled chicken breast
- 1 cup cherry tomatoes, halved
- 1 cucumber, diced
- 1/4 cup red onion, finely chopped
- 1/4 cup Kalamata olives, sliced
- 1/4 cup feta cheese, crumbled
- 2 tablespoons fresh parsley, chopped
- 2 tablespoons olive oil
- 1 tablespoon red wine vinegar
- 1 teaspoon dried oregano
- Salt and pepper to taste

Instructions:
1. In a pot, combine quinoa and water. Bring to a boil, then reduce heat and simmer for 15 minutes, or until water is absorbed and quinoa is tender. Let cool.
2. In a large bowl, combine cooked quinoa, grilled chicken, cherry tomatoes, cucumber, red onion, olives, feta cheese, and parsley.
3. In a small bowl, whisk together olive oil, red wine vinegar, oregano, salt, and pepper.
4. Pour the dressing over the salad and toss to combine.
5. Serve immediately or refrigerate for up to 3 days.

Nutritional Value (per serving):
Calories 350, Fat 14g, Carbohydrates 30g, Fiber 5g, Protein 25g, Sugars 6g, Sodium 550mg

Veggie-Packed Pasta Salad with Tuna

Prep Time: 15 minutes
Cooking Time: 10 minutes
Serving Size: 4

Ingredients:
- 8 oz whole grain pasta
- 1 can (5 oz) tuna in water, drained and flaked
- 1 cup cherry tomatoes, halved
- 1 cup cucumber, diced
- 1/2 cup bell pepper, diced
- 1/4 cup red onion, finely chopped
- 1/4 cup black olives, sliced
- 1/4 cup fresh basil, chopped
- 2 tablespoons olive oil
- 1 tablespoon lemon juice
- 1 teaspoon Dijon mustard
- Salt and pepper to taste

Instructions:
1. Cook the pasta according to package instructions. Drain and let cool.
2. In a large bowl, combine cooked pasta, tuna, cherry tomatoes, cucumber, bell pepper, red onion, olives, and basil.
3. In a small bowl, whisk together olive oil, lemon juice, Dijon mustard, salt, and pepper.
4. Pour the dressing over the salad and toss to combine.
5. Serve immediately or refrigerate for up to 3 days.

Nutritional Value (per serving):
Calories 300, Fat 10g, Carbohydrates 35g, Fiber 6g, Protein 18g, Sugars 5g, Sodium 450mg

Kale and Roasted Sweet Potato Salad with Tahini Dressing

Prep Time: 15 minutes
Cooking Time: 25 minutes
Serving Size: 4

Ingredients:
Salad:
- 1 large sweet potato, peeled and diced
- 1 tablespoon olive oil
- Salt and pepper to taste
- 1 bunch kale, stems removed and leaves chopped
- 1/4 cup dried cranberries
- 1/4 cup pumpkin seeds

Tahini Dressing:
- 1/4 cup tahini
- 2 tablespoons lemon juice
- 1 tablespoon maple syrup
- 1 clove garlic, minced
- 2-4 tablespoons water (to thin)
- Salt and pepper to taste

Instructions:
1. Preheat your oven to 400°F (200°C).
2. Toss the diced sweet potato with olive oil, salt, and pepper. Spread on a baking sheet and roast for 20-25 minutes, until tender and slightly browned.
3. In a large bowl, massage the chopped kale with a pinch of salt until it softens.
4. Add roasted sweet potatoes, dried cranberries, and pumpkin seeds to the kale.
5. In a small bowl, whisk together tahini, lemon juice, maple syrup, garlic, and water until smooth. Season with salt and pepper.
6. Drizzle the dressing over the salad and toss to combine.

Nutritional Value (per serving):
Calories 250, Fat 12g, Carbohydrates 32g, Fiber 7g, Protein 7g, Sugars 10g, Sodium 150mg

Grilled Salmon Nicoise Salad

Prep Time: 20 minutes
Cooking Time: 15 minutes
Serving Size: 4

Salad:
 - 4 salmon fillets (about 4 oz each)
 - 1 tablespoon olive oil
 - Salt and pepper to taste
 - 8 baby potatoes, halved
 - 2 cups green beans, trimmed
 - 4 hard-boiled eggs, halved
 - 1 cup cherry tomatoes, halved
 - 1/4 cup Kalamata olives

 - 4 cups mixed greens
Dressing:
 - 1/4 cup olive oil
 - 2 tablespoons lemon juice
 - 1 tablespoon Dijon mustard
 - 1 teaspoon honey
 - 1 clove garlic, minced
 - Salt and pepper to taste

1. Preheat your grill to medium-high heat. Brush the salmon fillets with olive oil and season with salt and pepper. Grill for 4-5 minutes per side, until cooked through. Let cool slightly.
2. Boil the baby potatoes until tender, about 10 minutes. In the last 2 minutes of cooking, add the green beans. Drain and set aside.
3. In a large bowl, combine mixed greens, potatoes, green beans, hard-boiled eggs, cherry tomatoes, and olives.
4. In a small bowl, whisk together olive oil, lemon juice, Dijon mustard, honey, and garlic. Season with salt and pepper.
5. Flake the grilled salmon into large pieces and add to the salad.
6. Drizzle the dressing over the salad and toss to combine.

 Calories 400, Fat 25g, Carbohydrates 20g, Fiber 6g, Protein 25g, Sugars 5g, Sodium 400mg

Southwestern Black Bean and Corn Salad

Prep Time: 15 minutes
Cooking Time: 0
Serving Size: 4

Ingredients:
- 1 can (15 oz) black beans, rinsed and drained
- 1 cup corn kernels (fresh or frozen)
- 1 red bell pepper, diced
- 1 avocado, diced
- 1/4 cup red onion, finely chopped
- 1/4 cup fresh cilantro, chopped
- 1/4 cup lime juice
- 2 tablespoons olive oil
- 1 teaspoon cumin
- 1/2 teaspoon chili powder
- Salt and pepper to taste

Instructions:
1. In a large bowl, combine black beans, corn, red bell pepper, avocado, red onion, and cilantro.
2. In a small bowl, whisk together lime juice, olive oil, cumin, chili powder, salt, and pepper.
3. Pour the dressing over the salad and toss to combine.
4. Serve immediately or refrigerate for up to 2 days.

Nutritional Value (per serving):
Calories 250, Fat 14g, Carbohydrates 28g, Fiber 10g, Protein 6g, Sugars 5g, Sodium 300mg

Asian-Inspired Chopped Salad with Edamame

Prep Time: 15 minutes
Cooking Time: 0
Serving Size: 4

Ingredients:

Salad:
- 2 cups Napa cabbage, shredded
- 1 cup red cabbage, shredded
- 1 cup carrots, shredded
- 1 cup edamame, shelled and cooked
- 1 red bell pepper, thinly sliced
- 1/4 cup green onions, chopped
- 1/4 cup fresh cilantro, chopped
- 1/4 cup roasted peanuts, chopped

Dressing:
- 1/4 cup rice vinegar
- 2 tablespoons soy sauce
- 1 tablespoon sesame oil
- 1 tablespoon honey
- 1 teaspoon grated fresh ginger
- 1 clove garlic, minced
- 1/4 teaspoon red pepper flakes (optional)

Instructions:

1. In a large bowl, combine Napa cabbage, red cabbage, carrots, edamame, red bell pepper, green onions, cilantro, and peanuts.
2. In a small bowl, whisk together rice vinegar, soy sauce, sesame oil, honey, ginger, garlic, and red pepper flakes, if using.
3. Pour the dressing over the salad and toss to combine.
4. Serve immediately or refrigerate for up to 2 days.

Nutritional Value (per serving):

Calories 200, Fat 10g, Carbohydrates 20g, Fiber 6g, Protein 8g, Sugars 8g, Sodium 400mg

Roasted Beet and Goat Cheese Salad with Walnuts

Prep Time: 15 minutes
Cooking Time: 45 minutes (for roasting beets)
Serving Size: 4

Ingredients:
Salad:
  - 4 medium beets, scrubbed and trimmed
  - 2 tablespoons olive oil
  - Salt and pepper to taste
  - 4 cups mixed greens
  - 1/4 cup goat cheese, crumbled
  - 1/4 cup walnuts, toasted and chopped
Dressing:
  - 1/4 cup balsamic vinegar
  - 2 tablespoons olive oil
  - 1 tablespoon honey
  - 1 teaspoon Dijon mustard
  - Salt and pepper to taste

Instructions:
1. Preheat your oven to 400°F (200°C). Wrap each beet in aluminum foil and place on a baking sheet. Roast for 45 minutes, or until tender. Let cool, then peel and dice.
2. In a large bowl, combine mixed greens, roasted beets, goat cheese, and walnuts.
3. In a small bowl, whisk together balsamic vinegar, olive oil, honey, Dijon mustard, salt, and pepper.
4. Pour the dressing over the salad and toss to combine.

Nutritional Value (per serving):
Calories 250, Fat 16g, Carbohydrates 22g, Fiber 6g, Protein 6g, Sugars 12g, Sodium 250mg

Creamy Cauliflower and White Bean Soup

Prep Time: 10 minutes
Cooking Time: 30 minutes
Serving Size: 4

Ingredients:
- 1 tablespoon olive oil
- 1 onion, diced
- 2 cloves garlic, minced
- 1 head cauliflower, chopped
- 1 can (15 oz) white beans, drained and rinsed
- 4 cups vegetable broth
- 1/2 cup unsweetened almond milk (or any milk of choice)
- 1 teaspoon thyme
- Salt and pepper to taste
- Fresh parsley, chopped (for garnish)

Instructions:

1. In a large pot, heat olive oil over medium heat. Add onion and garlic, sauté until softened.
2. Add cauliflower, white beans, vegetable broth, thyme, salt, and pepper. Bring to a boil, then reduce heat and simmer for 20 minutes, until cauliflower is tender.
3. Use an immersion blender to puree the soup until smooth. Alternatively, transfer to a blender in batches and blend until smooth.
4. Stir in almond milk and heat through.
5. Garnish with fresh parsley before serving.

Nutritional Value (per serving):

Calories 180, Fat 6g, Carbohydrates 25g, Fiber 8g, Protein 8g, Sugars 4g, Sodium 450mg

Turkey and Avocado Wrap with Sprouts

Prep Time: 10 minutes
Cooking Time: 0
Serving Size: 4

Ingredients:
- 4 large whole grain tortillas
- 8 slices deli turkey
- 2 avocados, sliced
- 1 cup alfalfa sprouts
- 1/2 cup shredded carrots
- 1/2 cup hummus
- Salt and pepper to taste

Instructions:
1. Lay out the tortillas and spread each with 2 tablespoons of hummus.
2. Layer with turkey slices, avocado slices, alfalfa sprouts, and shredded carrots.
3. Season with salt and pepper.
4. Roll up the tortillas tightly and slice in half.
5. Serve immediately or wrap and refrigerate for up to 1 day.

Nutritional Value (per serving):
 Calories 300, Fat 15g, Carbohydrates 30g, Fiber 8g, Protein 15g, Sugars 4g, Sodium 600mg

Lentil and Vegetable Minestrone

Prep Time: 15 minutes
Cooking Time: 30 minutes
Serving Size: 6

Ingredients:
- 1 tablespoon olive oil
- 1 onion, diced
- 2 cloves garlic, minced
- 2 carrots, diced
- 2 celery stalks, diced
- 1 zucchini, diced
- 1 can (15 oz) diced tomatoes
- 1 cup green or brown lentils, rinsed
- 6 cups vegetable broth
- 1 teaspoon dried oregano
- 1 teaspoon dried basil
- 1/2 teaspoon dried thyme
- 2 cups fresh spinach, chopped
- Salt and pepper to taste

Instructions:

1. In a large pot, heat olive oil over medium heat. Add onion, garlic, carrots, and celery, and sauté until softened.
2. Add zucchini and cook for another 2 minutes.
3. Stir in diced tomatoes, lentils, vegetable broth, oregano, basil, and thyme. Bring to a boil.
4. Reduce heat and simmer for 25-30 minutes, or until lentils are tender.
5. Stir in chopped spinach and cook until wilted.
6. Season with salt and pepper to taste.
7. Serve hot, garnished with fresh herbs if desired.

Nutritional Value (per serving):

Calories 200, Fat 4g, Carbohydrates 35g, Fiber 10g, Protein 10g, Sugars 8g, Sodium 500mg

Grilled Portobello Mushroom Sandwich with Pesto

Prep Time: 10 minutes
Cooking Time: 15 minutes
Serving Size: 4

Ingredients:

- 4 large portobello mushrooms, stems removed
- 2 tablespoons olive oil
- Salt and pepper to taste
- 4 whole grain sandwich rolls
- 1/2 cup pesto sauce
- 1 cup arugula
- 1 tomato, sliced
- 4 slices provolone cheese (optional)

Instructions:

1. Preheat grill or grill pan to medium-high heat.
2. Brush portobello mushrooms with olive oil and season with salt and pepper.
3. Grill mushrooms for 5-7 minutes on each side, until tender and slightly charred.
4. Toast sandwich rolls on the grill for 1-2 minutes, until lightly browned.
5. Spread pesto sauce on the bottom half of each roll.
6. Layer with grilled portobello mushrooms, arugula, tomato slices, and provolone cheese, if using.
7. Top with the other half of the roll and serve immediately.

Nutritional Value (per serving):

Calories 350, Fat 20g, Carbohydrates 30g, Fiber 6g, Protein 10g, Sugars 5g, Sodium 550mg

Butternut Squash and Apple Soup

Prep Time: 15 minutes
Cooking Time: 30 minutes
Serving Size: 4

Ingredients:
- 1 tablespoon olive oil
- 1 onion, diced
- 2 cloves garlic, minced
- 1 butternut squash, peeled, seeded, and diced
- 2 apples, peeled, cored, and diced
- 4 cups vegetable broth
- 1/2 teaspoon ground cinnamon
- 1/4 teaspoon ground nutmeg
- Salt and pepper to taste
- 1/2 cup coconut milk (optional, for creaminess)
- Fresh thyme for garnish (optional)

Instructions:

1. In a large pot, heat olive oil over medium heat. Add onion and garlic, and sauté until softened.
2. Add diced butternut squash and apples, cooking for another 5 minutes.
3. Pour in vegetable broth, cinnamon, nutmeg, salt, and pepper. Bring to a boil.
4. Reduce heat and simmer for 20-25 minutes, or until squash and apples are tender.
5. Use an immersion blender to puree the soup until smooth. Alternatively, transfer to a blender in batches and blend until smooth.
6. Stir in coconut milk, if using, and heat through.
7. Garnish with fresh thyme before serving.

Nutritional Value (per serving):

 Calories 220, Fat 8g, Carbohydrates 38g, Fiber 6g, Protein 3g, Sugars 18g, Sodium 400mg

Chapter 6: Dinner Recipes

One-Pan Lemon Herb Roasted Chicken with Vegetables

Prep Time: 15 minutes
Cooking Time: 45 minutes
Serving Size: 4

Ingredients:

- 4 bone-in, skin-on chicken thighs

- 1 lemon, sliced

- 3 cloves garlic, minced

- 2 tablespoons olive oil

- 1 teaspoon dried oregano

- 1 teaspoon dried thyme

- Salt and pepper to taste

- 4 cups mixed vegetables (potatoes, carrots, bell peppers, zucchini), chopped

Instructions:

1. Preheat your oven to 400°F (200°C).

2. In a large bowl, combine minced garlic, olive oil, dried oregano, dried thyme, salt, and pepper.

3. Add chicken thighs and mixed vegetables to the bowl, and toss to coat with the seasoning mixture.

4. Spread the chicken and vegetables on a large baking sheet in a single layer.

5. Place lemon slices on top of the chicken.

6. Roast in the oven for 40-45 minutes, or until the chicken is cooked through and the vegetables are tender and golden brown.

7. Serve hot, garnished with fresh herbs if desired.

Nutritional Value (per serving):

Calories 400, Fat 25g, Carbohydrates 20g, Fiber 5g, Protein 25g, Sugars 5g, Sodium 450mg

Slow Cooker Vegetarian Chili with Cornbread

Prep Time: 15 minutes
Cooking Time: 6-8 hours (slow cooker)
Serving Size: 6

Ingredients:
Chili:
- 1 tablespoon olive oil
- 1 onion, diced
- 2 cloves garlic, minced
- 1 bell pepper, diced
- 2 carrots, diced
- 1 zucchini, diced
- 1 can (15 oz) black beans, rinsed and drained
- 1 can (15 oz) kidney beans, rinsed and drained
- 1 can (15 oz) corn kernels, drained
- 1 can (28 oz) diced tomatoes
- 2 tablespoons chili powder
- 1 teaspoon cumin
- 1 teaspoon paprika
- Salt and pepper to taste

Cornbread:
- 1 cup cornmeal
- 1 cup all-purpose flour
- 1/4 cup sugar
- 1 tablespoon baking powder
- 1/2 teaspoon salt
- 1 cup milk
- 1/4 cup vegetable oil
- 1 large egg

1. In a large skillet, heat olive oil over medium heat. Add onion and garlic, sauté until softened.

2. Transfer the onion and garlic to a slow cooker. Add bell pepper, carrots, zucchini, black beans, kidney beans, corn, diced tomatoes, chili powder, cumin, paprika, salt, and pepper.

3. Stir to combine. Cover and cook on low for 6-8 hours or high for 3-4 hours.

4. Cornbread: Preheat your oven to 400°F (200°C). In a large bowl, combine cornmeal, flour, sugar, baking powder, and salt. In another bowl, whisk together milk, vegetable oil, and egg. Pour wet ingredients into dry ingredients and mix until just combined. Pour batter into a greased baking dish and bake for 20-25 minutes, or until a toothpick inserted into the center comes out clean.

5. Serve the chili hot, with a slice of cornbread on the side.

Nutritional Value (per serving, including cornbread):

Calories 450, Fat 15g, Carbohydrates 70g, Fiber 15g, Protein 15g, Sugars 15g, Sodium 600mg

Baked Salmon Cakes with Quinoa and Steamed Broccoli

Prep Time: 20 minutes
Cooking Time: 20 minutes
Serving Size: 4

Ingredients:

Salmon Cakes:
- 1 can (14 oz) salmon, drained and flaked
- 1/2 cup breadcrumbs
- 1/4 cup finely chopped onion
- 1/4 cup finely chopped bell pepper
- 1/4 cup mayonnaise
- 1 egg
- 1 tablespoon lemon juice
- 1 teaspoon Dijon mustard
- 1 teaspoon Old Bay seasoning

Quinoa:
- 1 cup quinoa, rinsed
- 2 cups water
- Steamed Broccoli:
- 4 cups broccoli florets
- Salt and pepper to taste
- Lemon wedges (for serving)

Instructions:

1. Salmon Cakes: Preheat your oven to 375°F (190°C). In a large bowl, combine salmon, breadcrumbs, onion, bell pepper, mayonnaise, egg, lemon juice, Dijon mustard, and Old Bay seasoning. Form the mixture into 8 patties and place them on a greased baking sheet. Bake for 15-20 minutes, or until golden brown.

2. Quinoa: In a pot, combine quinoa and water. Bring to a boil, then reduce heat and simmer for 15 minutes, or until water is absorbed and quinoa is tender. Fluff with a fork.

3. Steamed Broccoli: Steam broccoli florets until tender, about 5-7 minutes. Season with salt and pepper.

4. Serve salmon cakes with quinoa and steamed broccoli, garnished with lemon wedges.

Nutritional Value (per serving):

Calories 400, Fat 15g, Carbohydrates 40g, Fiber 8g, Protein 30g, Sugars 4g, Sodium 550mg

Turkey and Vegetable Lasagna

Prep Time: 30 minutes
Cooking Time: 1 hour
Serving Size: 8

Ingredients:

Lasagna:
- 12 lasagna noodles
- 1 tablespoon olive oil
- 1 onion, diced
- 2 cloves garlic, minced
- 1 pound ground turkey
- 2 cups spinach, chopped
- 2 cups ricotta cheese
- 1 egg
- 1/4 cup grated Parmesan cheese
- 4 cups marinara sauce
- 2 cups shredded mozzarella cheese
- Salt and pepper to taste

Instructions:

1. Preheat your oven to 375°F (190°C).
2. Cook lasagna noodles according to package instructions. Drain and set aside.
3. In a large skillet, heat olive oil over medium heat. Add onion and garlic, sauté until softened.
4. Add ground turkey and cook until browned. Stir in spinach and cook until wilted. Season with salt and pepper.
5. In a bowl, combine ricotta cheese, egg, and Parmesan cheese.
6. In a 9x13-inch baking dish, spread a thin layer of marinara sauce. Layer with 3 lasagna noodles, 1/3 of the turkey mixture, 1/3 of the ricotta mixture, and 1/3 of the shredded mozzarella. Repeat layers twice more, ending with a layer of marinara sauce and mozzarella cheese.
7. Cover with foil and bake for 45 minutes. Remove foil and bake for an additional 15 minutes, or until the cheese is golden and bubbly.
8. Let cool slightly before slicing and serving.

Nutritional Value (per serving):

Calories 450, Fat 20g, Carbohydrates 40g, Fiber 6g, Protein 30g, Sugars 8g, Sodium 700mg

Stir-Fried Tofu and Vegetable Noodle Bowl

Prep Time: 15 minutes
Cooking Time: 15 minutes
Serving Size: 4

Ingredients:
- 8 oz rice noodles
- 1 tablespoon sesame oil
- 1 block (14 oz) firm tofu, drained and cubed
- 1 red bell pepper, sliced
- 1 zucchini, sliced
- 1 cup snap peas
- 2 cloves garlic, minced
- 2 tablespoons soy sauce
- 1 tablespoon hoisin sauce
- 1 tablespoon rice vinegar
- 1 teaspoon grated fresh ginger
- 2 green onions, chopped
- Sesame seeds for garnish

Instructions:
1. Cook rice noodles according to package instructions. Drain and set aside.
2. In a large skillet or wok, heat sesame oil over medium-high heat. Add tofu and cook until golden brown on all sides. Remove from skillet and set aside.
3. In the same skillet, add red bell pepper, zucchini, and snap peas. Stir-fry for 3-4 minutes, until vegetables are tender-crisp.
4. Add garlic, soy sauce, hoisin sauce, rice vinegar, and ginger to the skillet. Stir to combine.
5. Return tofu to the skillet and add cooked noodles. Toss to combine and heat through.
6. Garnish with chopped green onions and sesame seeds before serving.

Nutritional Value (per serving):
Calories 350, Fat 12g, Carbohydrates 40g, Fiber 6g, Protein 15g, Sugars 6g, Sodium 600mg

Herb-Crusted Rack of Lamb with Roasted Root Vegetables

Prep Time: 20 minutes
Cooking Time: 35 minutes
Serving Size: 2

Ingredients:

Lamb:
- 1 rack of lamb (8 ribs)
- 2 tablespoons Dijon mustard
- 1/4 cup breadcrumbs
- 2 tablespoons fresh rosemary, chopped
- 2 tablespoons fresh thyme, chopped
- 2 cloves garlic, minced
- Salt and pepper to taste
- 2 tablespoons olive oil

Roasted Root Vegetables:
- 2 carrots, peeled and chopped
- 2 parsnips, peeled and chopped
- 1 sweet potato, peeled and chopped
- 1 tablespoon olive oil
- Salt and pepper to taste
- 1 teaspoon fresh thyme, chopped

Instructions:

1. Preheat your oven to 400°F (200°C).

2. Rub the lamb rack with Dijon mustard. In a small bowl, combine breadcrumbs, rosemary, thyme, garlic, salt, and pepper. Press the herb mixture onto the lamb rack.

3. In a large ovenproof skillet, heat olive oil over medium-high heat. Sear the lamb rack for 2-3 minutes on each side until browned.

4. Transfer the skillet to the oven and roast for 20-25 minutes for medium-rare, or until desired doneness. Let rest for 10 minutes before slicing.

5. Meanwhile, on a baking sheet, toss carrots, parsnips, and sweet potato with olive oil, salt, pepper, and thyme. Roast in the oven for 25-30 minutes, until tender and golden.

6. Serve the lamb chops with roasted root vegetables.

Nutritional Value (per serving):

Calories 700, Fat 45g, Carbohydrates 35g, Fiber 8g, Protein 40g, Sugars 10g, Sodium 600mg

Seared Scallops with Cauliflower Puree and Wilted Greens

Prep Time: 15 minutes
Cooking Time: 20 minutes
Serving Size: 2

Ingredients:

Scallops:
- 8 large sea scallops
- Salt and pepper to taste
- 1 tablespoon olive oil
- 1 tablespoon butter

Cauliflower Puree:
- 1 small head cauliflower, chopped
- 1/2 cup milk (or cream)
- 2 tablespoons butter
- Salt and pepper to taste

Wilted Greens:
- 2 cups baby spinach or mixed greens
- 1 tablespoon olive oil
- 1 clove garlic, minced
- Salt and pepper to taste

Instructions:

1. Cauliflower Puree: In a pot, bring cauliflower and milk to a boil. Reduce heat and simmer until cauliflower is tender, about 10 minutes. Drain, reserving some of the milk. Blend cauliflower with butter, salt, and pepper until smooth, adding reserved milk as needed for desired consistency. Keep warm.
2. Scallops: Pat scallops dry and season with salt and pepper. In a large skillet, heat olive oil and butter over medium-high heat. Sear scallops for 2-3 minutes on each side, until golden brown and cooked through. Remove from skillet and keep warm.
3. Wilted Greens: In the same skillet, heat olive oil over medium heat. Add garlic and cook until fragrant. Add spinach and cook until wilted. Season with salt and pepper.
4. Serve scallops on a bed of cauliflower puree, with wilted greens on the side.

Nutritional Value (per serving):

Calories 350, Fat 22g, Carbohydrates 20g, Fiber 6g, Protein 20g, Sugars 6g, Sodium 450mg

Stuffed Portobello Mushrooms with Spinach and Feta

Prep Time: 15 minutes
Cooking Time: 25 minutes
Serving Size: 2

Ingredients:

- 4 large portobello mushrooms, stems removed
- 2 tablespoons olive oil
- Salt and pepper to taste
- 1 small onion, diced
- 2 cloves garlic, minced
- 4 cups fresh spinach, chopped
- 1/2 cup feta cheese, crumbled
- 1/4 cup breadcrumbs
- 1 tablespoon fresh parsley, chopped

Instructions:

1. Preheat your oven to 375°F (190°C).
2. Brush portobello mushrooms with olive oil and season with salt and pepper. Place on a baking sheet, gill side up.
3. In a skillet, heat olive oil over medium heat. Add onion and garlic, sauté until softened. Add spinach and cook until wilted. Season with salt and pepper.
4. Remove from heat and stir in feta cheese, breadcrumbs, and parsley.
5. Spoon the spinach mixture into the mushroom caps.
6. Bake for 20-25 minutes, until mushrooms are tender and the filling is golden brown.
7. Serve hot, garnished with additional parsley if desired.

Nutritional Value (per serving):

Calories 300, Fat 20g, Carbohydrates 20g, Fiber 6g, Protein 10g, Sugars 5g, Sodium 600mg

Pan-Seared Duck Breast with Cherry Sauce and Wild Rice

Prep Time: 15 minutes
Cooking Time: 25 minutes
Serving Size: 2

Ingredients:
Duck:
 - 2 duck breasts
 - Salt and pepper to taste

Cherry Sauce:
 - 1 cup fresh or frozen cherries, pitted
 - 1/4 cup chicken broth
 - 1/4 cup red wine
 - 1 tablespoon balsamic vinegar
 - 1 tablespoon honey
 - 1 teaspoon cornstarch mixed with 1 tablespoon water

Wild Rice:
 - 1 cup wild rice
 - 2 cups water or chicken broth
 - 1 tablespoon butter
 - Salt and pepper to taste

Instructions:

1. Duck: Score the skin of the duck breasts in a crisscross pattern. Season with salt and pepper. In a cold skillet, place duck breasts skin side down. Cook over medium heat until the skin is crispy and brown, about 8-10 minutes. Flip and cook for another 5-6 minutes for medium-rare. Remove from skillet and let rest.

2. Cherry Sauce: In a small saucepan, combine cherries, chicken broth, red wine, balsamic vinegar, and honey. Bring to a boil, then reduce heat and simmer until cherries are soft. Stir in cornstarch mixture and cook until the sauce thickens.

3. Wild Rice: In a pot, combine wild rice and water (or chicken broth). Bring to a boil, then reduce heat and simmer for 20-25 minutes, until rice is tender. Stir in butter, salt, and pepper.

4. Serve duck breast sliced, drizzled with cherry sauce, and wild rice on the side.

Nutritional Value (per serving):

 Calories 600, Fat 30g, Carbohydrates 50g, Fiber 6g, Protein 30g, Sugars 15g, Sodium 450mg

Grilled Vegetable and Halloumi Skewers with Lemon Herb Couscous

Prep Time: 15 minutes
Cooking Time: 15 minutes
Serving Size: 2

Ingredients:

Skewers:
- 1 zucchini, sliced
- 1 red bell pepper, chopped
- 1 yellow bell pepper, chopped
- 8 cherry tomatoes
- 1 package halloumi cheese, cubed
- 2 tablespoons olive oil
- Salt and pepper to taste
- 1 teaspoon dried oregano

Lemon Herb Couscous:
- 1 cup couscous
- 1 cup vegetable broth
- 1 tablespoon olive oil
- 1 tablespoon lemon juice
- 1/4 cup fresh parsley, chopped
- 1/4 cup fresh mint, chopped
- Salt and pepper to taste

Instructions:

1. Skewers: Preheat grill to medium-high heat. Thread zucchini, bell peppers, cherry tomatoes, and halloumi cheese onto skewers. Brush with olive oil and season with salt, pepper, and oregano.
2. Grill skewers for 10-15 minutes, turning occasionally, until vegetables are tender and halloumi is golden brown.
3. Lemon Herb Couscous: In a pot, bring vegetable broth to a boil. Remove from heat and stir in couscous, olive oil, and lemon juice. Cover and let sit for 5 minutes, then fluff with a fork.
4. Stir in chopped parsley and mint, and season with salt and pepper.
5. Serve grilled vegetable and halloumi skewers over the lemon herb couscous.

Nutritional Value (per serving):

Calories 450, Fat 25g, Carbohydrates 40g, Fiber 6g, Protein 15g, Sugars 8g, Sodium 600mg

Spanish Seafood Paella

Prep Time: 20 minutes
Cooking Time: 40 minutes
Serving Size: 4

Ingredients:
- 2 tablespoons olive oil
- 1 onion, diced
- 3 cloves garlic, minced
- 1 red bell pepper, diced
- 1 cup Arborio rice
- 1/2 teaspoon smoked paprika
- 1/4 teaspoon saffron threads
- 1/2 cup white wine
- 3 cups chicken broth
- 1 cup diced tomatoes
- 1/2 pound shrimp, peeled and deveined
- 1/2 pound mussels, cleaned
- 1/2 pound clams, cleaned
- 1/2 cup frozen peas
- 1 lemon, cut into wedges
- Fresh parsley, chopped (for garnish)
- Salt and pepper to taste

Instructions:

1. In a large skillet or paella pan, heat olive oil over medium heat. Add onion, garlic, and red bell pepper, sauté until softened.
2. Stir in Arborio rice, smoked paprika, and saffron. Cook for 1-2 minutes until rice is lightly toasted.
3. Add white wine, cooking until it evaporates. Stir in chicken broth and diced tomatoes, bringing to a simmer.
4. Cook for 15 minutes, stirring occasionally, until rice is almost tender.
5. Add shrimp, mussels, clams, and peas. Cover and cook for 5-7 minutes, or until seafood is cooked and mussels and clams have opened.
6. Season with salt and pepper. Garnish with lemon wedges and fresh parsley before serving.

Nutritional Value (per serving):

Calories 400, Fat 12g, Carbohydrates 45g, Fiber 5g, Protein 25g, Sugars 6g, Sodium 800mg

Moroccan-Spiced Chickpea and Vegetable Tagine

Prep Time: 15 minutes
Cooking Time: 30 minutes
Serving Size: 4

Ingredients:

- 2 tablespoons olive oil
- 1 onion, diced
- 3 cloves garlic, minced
- 2 carrots, diced
- 1 zucchini, diced
- 1 red bell pepper, diced
- 1 can (15 oz) chickpeas, drained and rinsed
- 1 can (14.5 oz) diced tomatoes
- 1/2 cup dried apricots, chopped
- 1 teaspoon ground cumin
- 1 teaspoon ground cinnamon
- 1 teaspoon ground turmeric
- 1/2 teaspoon ground ginger
- 1/2 teaspoon ground paprika
- 2 cups vegetable broth
- 1/4 cup fresh cilantro, chopped (for garnish)
- Salt and pepper to taste
- Cooked couscous (for serving)

Instructions:

1. In a large pot or tagine, heat olive oil over medium heat. Add onion and garlic, sauté until softened.
2. Add carrots, zucchini, and red bell pepper. Cook for 5 minutes until vegetables begin to soften.
3. Stir in chickpeas, diced tomatoes, dried apricots, cumin, cinnamon, turmeric, ginger, and paprika. Cook for 1-2 minutes until fragrant.
4. Add vegetable broth, bringing to a simmer. Cook for 20 minutes until vegetables are tender.
5. Season with salt and pepper. Garnish with fresh cilantro and serve with cooked couscous.

Nutritional Value (per serving):

Calories 350, Fat 10g, Carbohydrates 60g, Fiber 15g, Protein 10g, Sugars 20g, Sodium 500mg

Coconut Curry Lentil Soup with Sweet Potatoes

Prep Time: 15 minutes
Cooking Time: 30 minutes
Serving Size: 4

Ingredients:
- 1 tablespoon coconut oil
- 1 onion, diced
- 3 cloves garlic, minced
- 1 tablespoon ginger, minced
- 1 tablespoon curry powder
- 1 teaspoon ground cumin
- 1/2 teaspoon ground turmeric
- 1 sweet potato, peeled and diced
- 1 cup red lentils, rinsed
- 1 can (14 oz) coconut milk
- 4 cups vegetable broth
- 2 cups baby spinach
- Salt and pepper to taste
- Fresh cilantro, chopped (for garnish)
- Lime wedges (for serving)

Instructions:
1. In a large pot, heat coconut oil over medium heat. Add onion, garlic, and ginger, sauté until softened.
2. Stir in curry powder, cumin, and turmeric, cooking for 1-2 minutes until fragrant.
3. Add sweet potato, red lentils, coconut milk, and vegetable broth. Bring to a boil, then reduce heat and simmer for 20-25 minutes until lentils and sweet potatoes are tender.
4. Stir in baby spinach until wilted. Season with salt and pepper.
5. Garnish with fresh cilantro and serve with lime wedges.

Nutritional Value (per serving):
 Calories 350, Fat 15g, Carbohydrates 45g, Fiber 12g, Protein 10g, Sugars 8g, Sodium 600mg

One-Pot Chicken and Mushroom Wild Rice Casserole

Prep Time: 15 minutes
Cooking Time: 45 minutes
Serving Size: 4

Ingredients:
- 1 tablespoon olive oil
- 1 pound chicken breasts, cut into bite-sized pieces
- Salt and pepper to taste
- 1 onion, diced
- 2 cloves garlic, minced
- 2 cups mushrooms, sliced
- 1 cup wild rice
- 3 cups chicken broth
- 1/2 cup heavy cream
- 1/4 cup grated Parmesan cheese
- 1/4 cup fresh parsley, chopped (for garnish)

Instructions:
1. In a large pot, heat olive oil over medium-high heat. Season chicken with salt and pepper. Cook chicken until browned, then remove from pot and set aside.
2. In the same pot, add onion, garlic, and mushrooms, sauté until softened.
3. Stir in wild rice and chicken broth. Bring to a boil, then reduce heat, cover, and simmer for 35-40 minutes until rice is tender.
4. Stir in heavy cream and cooked chicken, cooking until heated through.
5. Sprinkle with Parmesan cheese and garnish with fresh parsley before serving.

Nutritional Value (per serving):
Calories 450, Fat 20g, Carbohydrates 35g, Fiber 5g, Protein 30g, Sugars 4g, Sodium 600mg

Vegetarian Stuffed Bell Peppers with Quinoa and Black Beans

Prep Time: 15 minutes
Cooking Time: 40 minutes
Serving Size: 4

Ingredients:

- 4 large bell peppers, tops cut off and seeds removed
- 1 tablespoon olive oil
- 1 onion, diced
- 2 cloves garlic, minced
- 1 cup cooked quinoa
- 1 can (15 oz) black beans, drained and rinsed
- 1 cup corn kernels (fresh or frozen)
- 1 can (14.5 oz) diced tomatoes
- 1 teaspoon ground cumin
- 1 teaspoon chili powder
- Salt and pepper to taste
- 1 cup shredded cheddar cheese (optional)
- Fresh cilantro, chopped (for garnish)

Instructions:

1. Preheat your oven to 375°F (190°C).
2. In a large skillet, heat olive oil over medium heat. Add onion and garlic, sauté until softened.
3. Stir in cooked quinoa, black beans, corn, diced tomatoes, cumin, chili powder, salt, and pepper. Cook for 5 minutes until heated through.
4. Stuff each bell pepper with the quinoa mixture and place them in a baking dish. Top with shredded cheddar cheese, if using.
5. Cover with foil and bake for 30 minutes. Remove foil and bake for an additional 10 minutes until peppers are tender and cheese is melted.
6. Garnish with fresh cilantro before serving.

Nutritional Value (per serving):

Calories 350, Fat 12g, Carbohydrates 50g, Fiber 12g, Protein 12g, Sugars 8g, Sodium 500mg

Chapter 7: Smoothies and Beverages

Green Goddess Smoothie

Prep Time: 5 minutes
Serving Size: 1

Ingredients:
- 1 cup spinach
- 1/2 avocado
- 1 banana
- 1 cup almond milk
- 1 tablespoon chia seeds

Instructions:
Blend all ingredients until smooth and enjoy!

Nutritional Value (per serving):
Calories: 250
Fat: 15g
Carbohydrates: 30g
Fiber: 10g
Protein: 5g
Sugars: 6g

Berry and Flaxseed Boost

Prep Time: 5 minutes
Serving Size: 1

Ingredients:
- 1 cup mixed berries (fresh or frozen)
- 1 tablespoon flaxseeds
- 1 cup yogurt (dairy or plant-based)
- 1 teaspoon honey (optional)

Instructions:
Blend until creamy and serve chilled.

Nutritional Value (per serving):
Calories: 200
Fat: 5g
Carbohydrates: 30g
Fiber: 8g
Protein: 8g
Sugars: 10g

Maca and Cacao Energizer

Prep Time: 5 minutes
Serving Size: 1

Ingredients:
- 1 tablespoon maca powder
- 1 tablespoon cacao powder
- 1 banana
- 1 cup coconut milk
- 1 tablespoon almond butter

Instructions:
Blend until smooth and enjoy the rich flavor!

Nutritional Value (per serving):
Calories: 350
Fat: 20g
Carbohydrates: 40g
Fiber: 6g
Protein: 8g
Sugars: 10g

Tropical Turmeric Bliss

Prep Time: 5 minutes
Serving Size: 1

Ingredients:
- 1 cup pineapple chunks
- 1/2 banana
- 1 teaspoon turmeric powder
- 1 cup coconut water
- 1 tablespoon ginger (fresh or powdered)

Instructions:
Blend until well combined for a refreshing taste.

Nutritional Value (per serving):
Calories: 150
Fat: 1g
Carbohydrates: 35g
Fiber: 4g
Protein: 2g
Sugars: 25g

Creamy Avocado and Spinach Smoothie

Prep Time: 5 minutes
Serving Size: 1

Ingredients:
- 1/2 avocado
- 1 cup spinach
- 1 cup almond milk
- 1 tablespoon lemon juice
- 1 tablespoon honey (optional)

Instructions:
Blend until creamy and enjoy the nutrients!

Nutritional Value (per serving):
Calories: 230
Fat: 15g
Carbohydrates: 20g
Fiber: 7g
Protein: 5g
Sugars: 8g

Herbal Teas for Women's Health

Red Clover and Nettle Infusion

Prep Time: 5 minutes
Steeping Time: 10-15 minutes
Serving Size: 1 cup

Ingredients:
- 1 teaspoon dried red clover flowers
- 1 teaspoon dried nettle leaves
- 1 cup boiling water

Instructions:
1. Combine the herbs in a tea infuser or teapot.
2. Pour boiling water over the herbs and steep for 10-15 minutes.
3. Strain and enjoy!

Nutritional Value (per cup):
Calories: 5
Fat: 0g
Carbohydrates: 1g
Protein: 0g

Calming Chamomile and Lavender Blend

Prep Time: 5 minutes
Steeping Time: 5-10 minutes
Serving Size: 1 cup

Ingredients:

- 1 tablespoon dried chamomile flowers
- 1 teaspoon dried lavender flowers
- 1 cup boiling water

Instructions:

1. Combine chamomile and lavender in a tea infuser.
2. Pour boiling water over the herbs and steep for 5-10 minutes.
3. Strain and savor the calming effect!

Nutritional Value (per cup):

Calories: 5
Fat: 0g
Carbohydrates: 1g
Protein: 0g

Vitex Berry Balance Tea

Prep Time: 5 minutes
Steeping Time: 10-15 minutes
Serving Size: 1 cup

Ingredients:
- 1 teaspoon dried vitex (chaste tree) berries
- 1 cup boiling water

Instructions:
1. Crush the vitex berries slightly and place in a tea infuser.
2. Pour boiling water over and steep for 10-15 minutes.
3. Strain and enjoy!

Nutritional Value (per cup):
Calories: 5
Fat: 0g
Carbohydrates: 1g
Protein: 0g

Ginger and Cinnamon Digestive Aid

Prep Time: 5 minutes
Steeping Time: 10 minutes
Serving Size: 1 cup

Ingredients:

- 1 teaspoon fresh ginger, grated
- 1/2 teaspoon cinnamon powder
- 1 cup boiling water

Instructions:

1. Combine ginger and cinnamon in a cup.
2. Pour boiling water over the mixture and steep for 10 minutes.
3. Strain and enjoy the warming effects!

Nutritional Value (per cup):
Calories: 10
Fat: 0g
Carbohydrates: 3g
Protein: 0g

Raspberry Leaf and Peppermint Tonic

Prep Time: 5 minutes
Steeping Time: 10-15 minutes
Serving Size: 1 cup

Ingredients:
- 1 tablespoon dried raspberry leaf
- 1 teaspoon dried peppermint leaves
- 1 cup boiling water

Instructions:
1. Combine raspberry leaf and peppermint in a tea infuser.
2. Pour boiling water over the herbs and steep for 10-15 minutes.
3. Strain and enjoy the refreshing taste!

Nutritional Value (per cup):
Calories: 5
Fat: 0g
Carbohydrates: 1g
Protein: 0g

Infused Waters

Cucumber, Lemon, and Mint Refresher

Prep Time: 5 minutes
Infusion Time: 2 hours
Serving Size: 1 pitcher

Ingredients:
- 1 cucumber, sliced
- 1 lemon, sliced
- A handful of fresh mint leaves
- 8 cups water

Instructions:
1. Combine cucumber, lemon, and mint in a pitcher.
2. Add water and refrigerate for at least 2 hours.
3. Serve chilled!

Nutritional Value (per serving):
Calories: 5
Fat: 0g
Carbohydrates: 1g
Protein: 0g

Strawberry and Basil Elixir

Prep Time: 5 minutes
Infusion Time: 2 hours
Serving Size: 1 pitcher

Ingredients:

- 1 cup strawberries, hulled and sliced
- A handful of fresh basil leaves
- 8 cups water

Instructions:

1. Combine strawberries and basil in a pitcher.
2. Add water and refrigerate for at least 2 hours.
3. Serve chilled!

Nutritional Value (per serving):

Calories: 10
Fat: 0g
Carbohydrates: 2g
Protein: 0g

Ginger, Turmeric, and Orange Zest Water

Prep Time: 5 minutes
Infusion Time: 2 hours
Serving Size: 1 pitcher

Ingredients:
- 1-inch fresh ginger, sliced
- 1-inch fresh turmeric, sliced (or 1 teaspoon turmeric powder)
- Zest of 1 orange
- 8 cups water

Instructions:
1. Combine ginger, turmeric, and orange zest in a pitcher.
2. Add water and refrigerate for at least 2 hours.
3. Serve chilled!

Nutritional Value (per serving):
Calories: 5
Fat: 0g
Carbohydrates: 1g
Protein: 0g

Rosemary and Grapefruit Infusion

Prep Time: 5 minutes
Infusion Time: 2 hours
Serving Size: 1 pitcher

Ingredients:

- 2 sprigs fresh rosemary
- 1 grapefruit, sliced
- 8 cups water

Instructions:

1. Combine rosemary and grapefruit in a pitcher.
2. Add water and refrigerate for at least 2 hours.
3. Serve chilled!

Nutritional Value (per serving):

Calories: 5
Fat: 0g
Carbohydrates: 1g
Protein: 0g

Blueberry and Sage Hydrator

Prep Time: 5 minutes
Infusion Time: 2 hours
Serving Size: 1 pitcher

Ingredients:
- 1 cup fresh blueberries
- A handful of fresh sage leaves
- 8 cups water

Instructions:
1. Combine blueberries and sage in a pitcher.
2. Add water and refrigerate for at least 2 hours.
3. Serve chilled!

Nutritional Value (per serving):
Calories: 10
Fat: 0g
Carbohydrates: 2g
Protein: 0g

Chapter 8: Snacks and Desserts

Roasted Chickpea Trail Mix

Prep Time: 10 minutes
Cooking Time: 30 minutes
Serving Size: 4

Ingredients:
- 1 can (15 oz) chickpeas, rinsed and drained
- 1 tablespoon olive oil
- 1 teaspoon garlic powder
- 1 teaspoon paprika
- Salt to taste

Instructions:
1. Preheat oven to 400°F (200°C).
2. Toss chickpeas with olive oil and seasonings.
3. Spread on a baking sheet and roast for 30 minutes until crispy.

Nutritional Value (per serving):
Calories: 150
Fat: 5g
Carbohydrates: 22g
Protein: 7g
Fiber: 6g

Vegetable Crudités with Hummus

Prep Time: 10 minutes
Serving Size: 4

Ingredients:

- Assorted vegetables (carrots, celery, bell peppers, cucumber)
- 1 cup hummus

Instructions:

1. Cut vegetables into sticks.
2. Serve with hummus for dipping.

Nutritional Value (per serving):

Calories: 100
Fat: 4g
Carbohydrates: 14g
Protein: 3g
Fiber: 4g

Apple Slices with Almond Butter

Prep Time: 5 minutes
Serving Size: 1

Ingredients:
- 1 apple, sliced
- 2 tablespoons almond butter

Instructions:
1. Slice the apple and serve with almond butter for dipping.

Nutritional Value (per serving):
Calories: 200
Fat: 10g
Carbohydrates: 26g
Protein: 4g
Fiber: 5g

Edamame with Sea Salt

Prep Time: 5 minutes
Cooking Time: 5 minutes
Serving Size: 1 cup

Ingredients:
- 1 cup shelled edamame
- Sea salt to taste

Instructions:
1. Boil or steam edamame for 5 minutes.
2. Sprinkle with sea salt and enjoy!

Nutritional Value (per serving):
Calories: 120
Fat: 5g
Carbohydrates: 10g
Protein: 11g
Fiber: 6g

Homemade Kale Chips

Prep Time: 10 minutes
Cooking Time: 15 minutes
Serving Size: 4

Ingredients:

- 1 bunch kale, torn into pieces
- 1 tablespoon olive oil
- Salt to taste

Instructions:

1. Preheat oven to 350°F (175°C).
2. Toss kale with olive oil and salt.
3. Spread on a baking sheet and bake for 15 minutes until crispy.

Nutritional Value (per serving):

Calories: 50
Fat: 3g
Carbohydrates: 7g
Protein: 2g
Fiber: 2g

Chia Seed Pudding with Berries

Prep Time: 10 minutes
Chilling Time: 2 hours
Serving Size: 2

Ingredients:
- 1/2 cup chia seeds
- 2 cups almond milk
- 1 tablespoon maple syrup (optional)
- 1 cup mixed berries

Instructions:
1. Mix chia seeds, almond milk, and maple syrup in a bowl.
2. Refrigerate for at least 2 hours until thickened.
3. Top with berries before serving.

Nutritional Value (per serving):
Calories: 200
Fat: 10g
Carbohydrates: 25g
Protein: 6g
Fiber: 12g

Baked Cinnamon Apples

Prep Time: 5 minutes
Cooking Time: 20 minutes
Serving Size: 4

Ingredients:
- 4 apples, cored and sliced
- 1 teaspoon cinnamon
- 1 tablespoon honey (optional)

Instructions:
1. Preheat oven to 350°F (175°C).
2. Toss apples with cinnamon and honey.
3. Bake for 20 minutes until soft.

Nutritional Value (per serving):
Calories: 120
Fat: 0g
Carbohydrates: 32g
Protein: 1g
Fiber: 5g

Dark Chocolate Avocado Mousse

Prep Time: 10 minutes
Chilling Time: 30 minutes
Serving Size: 2

Ingredients:
- 1 ripe avocado
- 1/4 cup cocoa powder
- 1/4 cup maple syrup
- 1 teaspoon vanilla extract

Instructions:
1. Blend all ingredients until smooth.
2. Refrigerate for 30 minutes before serving.

Nutritional Value (per serving):
Calories: 180
Fat: 10g
Carbohydrates: 24g
Protein: 3g
Fiber: 6g

Greek Yogurt Parfait with Honey and Walnuts

Prep Time: 5 minutes
Serving Size: 1

Ingredients:
- 1 cup Greek yogurt
- 1 tablespoon honey
- 1/4 cup walnuts, chopped
- Fresh fruit (optional)

Instructions:
1. Layer Greek yogurt, honey, and walnuts in a bowl.
2. Top with fresh fruit if desired.

Nutritional Value (per serving):
Calories: 300
Fat: 15g
Carbohydrates: 25g
Protein: 15g
Fiber: 2g

Grilled Peaches with Vanilla Cashew Cream

Prep Time: 5 minutes
Cooking Time: 10 minutes
Serving Size: 4

Ingredients:
- 4 peaches, halved and pitted
- 1 cup cashews (soaked)
- 1 teaspoon vanilla extract
- 1 tablespoon maple syrup (optional)

Instructions:
1. Preheat grill to medium heat.
2. Grill peach halves for about 5 minutes until charred.
3. Blend-soaked cashews, vanilla, and maple syrup until creamy.
4. Serve grilled peaches topped with cashew cream.

Nutritional Value (per serving):
Calories: 250
Fat: 15g
Carbohydrates: 30g
Protein: 5g
Fiber: 4g

Almond Joy Energy Balls

Prep Time: 10 minutes
Chilling Time: 30 minutes
Serving Size: 12

Ingredients:
- 1 cup dates, pitted
- 1 cup almond butter
- 1 cup shredded coconut
- 1/4 cup cocoa powder
- 1/2 cup almonds, chopped

Instructions:
1. In a food processor, blend dates and almond butter until smooth.
2. Add coconut, cocoa powder, and chopped almonds, and mix until combined.
3. Roll into bite-sized balls and chill for 30 minutes.

Nutritional Value (per ball):
Calories: 150
Fat: 10g
Carbohydrates: 15g
Protein: 3g
Fiber: 3g

Pumpkin Spice Protein Bites

Prep Time: 10 minutes
Chilling Time: 30 minutes
Serving Size: 12

Ingredients:
- 1 cup pumpkin puree
- 1 cup oats
- 1/2 cup protein powder
- 1 teaspoon pumpkin spice
- 1/4 cup maple syrup

Instructions:
1. In a bowl, combine pumpkin puree, oats, protein powder, pumpkin spice, and maple syrup.
2. Mix until well combined, then roll into balls.
3. Chill for 30 minutes before serving.

Nutritional Value (per bite):
Calories: 100
Fat: 2g
Carbohydrates: 18g
Protein: 5g
Fiber: 3g

Matcha Green Tea Energy Bars

Prep Time: 15 minutes
Chilling Time: 2 hours
Serving Size: 10

Ingredients:

- 1 cup oats
- 1/2 cup almond butter
- 1/4 cup honey
- 2 tablespoons matcha powder
- 1/4 cup chia seeds

Instructions:

1. In a bowl, mix all ingredients until well combined.

2. Press mixture into a lined baking dish and refrigerate for 2 hours.

3. Cut into bars and enjoy!

Nutritional Value (per bar):

Calories: 180

Fat: 8g

Carbohydrates: 24g

Protein: 6g

Fiber: 5g

Coconut and Goji Berry Bliss Balls

Prep Time: 10 minutes
Chilling Time: 30 minutes
Serving Size: 12

Ingredients:
- 1 cup dates, pitted
- 1/2 cup shredded coconut
- 1/2 cup goji berries
- 1/4 cup almond flour
- 1 tablespoon coconut oil

Instructions:
1. Blend dates and coconut oil in a food processor until smooth.
2. Add shredded coconut, goji berries, and almond flour, mixing until combined.
3. Roll into balls and chill for 30 minutes.

Nutritional Value (per ball):
Calories: 120
Fat: 5g
Carbohydrates: 20g
Protein: 2g
Fiber: 4g

Carrot Cake Protein Squares

Prep Time: 15 minutes
Chilling Time: 1 hour
Serving Size: 12

Ingredients:
- 1 cup grated carrots
- 1 cup oats
- 1/2 cup protein powder
- 1/4 cup almond butter
- 1 teaspoon cinnamon
- 1/4 cup maple syrup

Instructions:
1. In a bowl, combine grated carrots, oats, protein powder, almond butter, cinnamon, and maple syrup.
2. Mix until well combined and press into a lined baking dish.
3. Chill for 1 hour and cut into squares.

Nutritional Value (per square):
Calories: 150
Fat: 6g
Carbohydrates: 20g
Protein: 5g
Fiber: 3g

Chapter 9: 21-day Meal Plan

Day 1:

Breakfast: Overnight Chia Seed Pudding
Lunch: Lentil and Roasted Vegetable Grain Bowl
Dinner: One-Pan Lemon Herb Roasted Chicken with Vegetables
Smoothie: Green Goddess Smoothie
Snack: Roasted Chickpea Trail Mix

Day 2:

Breakfast: Spinach and Feta Egg Muffins
Lunch: Mediterranean Quinoa Salad with Grilled Chicken
Dinner: Slow Cooker Vegetarian Chili with Cornbread
Tea: Red Clover and Nettle Infusion
Dessert: Baked Cinnamon Apples

Day 3:

Breakfast: Avocado Toast with Smoked Salmon
Lunch: Kale and Roasted Sweet Potato Salad with Tahini Dressing
Dinner: Baked Salmon Cakes with Quinoa and Steamed Broccoli
Smoothie: Berry and Flaxseed Boost
Snack: Apple Slices with Almond Butter

Day 4:

Breakfast: Greek Yogurt Parfait with Berries and Flaxseeds
Lunch: Creamy Cauliflower and White Bean Soup
Dinner: Turkey and Vegetable Lasagna
Infused Water: Cucumber, Lemon, and Mint Refresher
Dessert: Dark Chocolate Avocado Mousse

Day 5:

Breakfast: Whole Grain Breakfast Smoothie Bowl
Lunch: Chickpea Salad Stuffed Pita Pockets
Dinner: Stir-Fried Tofu and Vegetable Noodle Bowl
Tea: Calming Chamomile and Lavender Blend
Snack: Edamame with Sea Salt

Day 6:
Breakfast: Quinoa Vegetable Frittata
Lunch: Grilled Salmon Nicoise Salad
Dinner: Herb-Crusted Rack of Lamb with Roasted Root Vegetables
Smoothie: Maca and Cacao Energizer
Energy Bite: Almond Joy Energy Balls

Day 7:
Breakfast: Buckwheat Pancakes with Blueberry Compote
Lunch: Turkey and Avocado Wrap with Sprouts
Dinner: Spanish Seafood Paella
Infused Water: Strawberry and Basil Elixir
Dessert: Greek Yogurt Parfait with Honey and Walnuts

Day 8:
Breakfast: Shakshuka with Whole Grain Pita
Lunch: Southwestern Black Bean and Corn Salad
Dinner: Seared Scallops with Cauliflower Puree and Wilted Greens
Tea: Vitex Berry Balance Tea
Snack: Homemade Kale Chips

Day 9:
Breakfast: Sweet Potato and Black Bean Breakfast Burrito
Lunch: Asian-Inspired Chopped Salad with Edamame
Dinner: Moroccan-Spiced Chickpea and Vegetable Tagine
Smoothie: Tropical Turmeric Bliss
Energy Bite: Pumpkin Spice Protein Bites

Day 10:
Breakfast: Smoked Tofu and Vegetable Scramble
Lunch: Lentil and Vegetable Minestrone
Dinner: Stuffed Portobello Mushrooms with Spinach and Feta
Infused Water: Ginger, Turmeric, and Orange Zest Water
Dessert: Chia Seed Pudding with Berries

Day 11:

Breakfast: Baked Oatmeal Cups with Apples and Walnuts
Lunch: Roasted Beet and Goat Cheese Salad with Walnuts
Dinner: Pan-Seared Duck Breast with Cherry Sauce and Wild Rice
Tea: Ginger and Cinnamon Digestive Aid
Snack: Vegetable Crudités with Hummus

Day 12:

Breakfast: Veggie-Packed Breakfast Casserole
Lunch: Grilled Portobello Mushroom Sandwich with Pesto
Dinner: Coconut Curry Lentil Soup with Sweet Potatoes
Smoothie: Creamy Avocado and Spinach Smoothie
Energy Bite: Matcha Green Tea Energy Bars

Day 13:

Breakfast: Protein-Rich Breakfast Cookies
Lunch: Butternut Squash and Apple Soup
Dinner: Grilled Vegetable and Halloumi Skewers with Lemon Herb Couscous
Infused Water: Rosemary and Grapefruit Infusion
Dessert: Grilled Peaches with Vanilla Cashew Cream

Day 14:

Breakfast: Mason Jar Layered Greek Yogurt Parfaits
Lunch: Sesame Ginger Tofu Lettuce Wraps
Dinner: One-Pot Chicken and Mushroom Wild Rice Casserole
Tea: Raspberry Leaf and Peppermint Tonic
Snack: Roasted Chickpea Trail Mix

Day 15:

Breakfast: Freezer-Friendly Breakfast Burritos
Lunch: Veggie-Packed Pasta Salad with Tuna
Dinner: Vegetarian Stuffed Bell Peppers with Quinoa and Black Beans
Smoothie: Green Goddess Smoothie
Energy Bite: Coconut and Goji Berry Bliss Balls

Day 16:

Breakfast: Overnight Chia Seed Pudding

Lunch: Mediterranean Quinoa Salad with Grilled Chicken

Dinner: One-Pan Lemon Herb Roasted Chicken with Vegetables

Infused Water: Blueberry and Sage Hydrator

Dessert: Baked Cinnamon Apples

Day 17:

Breakfast: Spinach and Feta Egg Muffins

Lunch: Kale and Roasted Sweet Potato Salad with Tahini Dressing

Dinner: Slow Cooker Vegetarian Chili with Cornbread

Tea: Red Clover and Nettle Infusion

Snack: Apple Slices with Almond Butter

Day 18:

Breakfast: Avocado Toast with Smoked Salmon

Lunch: Creamy Cauliflower and White Bean Soup

Dinner: Baked Salmon Cakes with Quinoa and Steamed Broccoli

Smoothie: Berry and Flaxseed Boost

Energy Bite: Carrot Cake Protein Squares

Day 19:

Breakfast: Greek Yogurt Parfait with Berries and Flaxseeds

Lunch: Chickpea Salad Stuffed Pita Pockets

Dinner: Turkey and Vegetable Lasagna

Infused Water: Cucumber, Lemon, and Mint Refresher

Dessert: Dark Chocolate Avocado Mousse

Day 20:

Breakfast: Whole Grain Breakfast Smoothie Bowl

Lunch: Grilled Salmon Nicoise Salad

Dinner: Stir-Fried Tofu and Vegetable Noodle Bowl

Tea: Calming Chamomile and Lavender Blend

Snack: Edamame with Sea Salt

Breakfast: Quinoa Vegetable Frittata
Lunch: Turkey and Avocado Wrap with Sprouts
Dinner: Spanish Seafood Paella
Smoothie: Maca and Cacao Energizer
Dessert: Greek Yogurt Parfait with Honey and Walnuts

Customizable Shopping Lists

To create a customizable shopping list, categorize ingredients by food groups and store sections. Here's a template:

Produce:

- (List vegetables and fruits needed for the week)

Proteins:

- (List meats, fish, tofu, eggs, etc.)

Dairy and Alternatives:

- (List milk, yogurt, cheese, plant-based alternatives)

Grains and Legumes:

- (List whole grains, beans, lentils, etc.)

Nuts and Seeds:

- (List various nuts and seeds)

Herbs and Spices:

- (List fresh herbs and dried spices)

Pantry Items:

- (List canned goods, oils, vinegars, etc.)

Frozen Foods:

- (List any frozen fruits, vegetables, or prepared items)

Other:

- (List any miscellaneous items)

Tips for Budget-Friendly Shopping:

1. Plan meals around seasonal produce, which is often cheaper and more nutritious.

2. Buy in bulk for non-perishable items and frequently used ingredients.

3. Choose frozen fruits and vegetables when fresh options are expensive.

4. Opt for less expensive protein sources like eggs, legumes, and canned fish.

5. Use cheaper cuts of meat for slow-cooker recipes.

6. Buy whole foods rather than pre-cut or prepared items.

7. Compare unit prices to get the best value.

8. Use store brands for staple items.

9. Shop at farmers markets, especially near closing time for potential discounts.

10. Grow your own herbs in small pots or a garden.

11. Use apps or websites to compare prices across different stores.

12. Buy generic or store-brand versions of pantry staples.

13. Look for markdowns on soon-to-expire items, especially for ingredients you'll use quickly.

14. Join store loyalty programs for discounts and personalized coupons.

15. Meal plan around store sales and promotions.

Methods to Preserve Nutrients

1. Steam Cooking:

Steaming vegetables helps retain water-soluble vitamins and minerals. Use a steamer basket or microwave steaming to preserve nutrients while achieving a tender texture.

2. Quick Sautéing:

Briefly cooking vegetables in a small amount of healthy oil over high heat preserves nutrients while enhancing flavor. Use this method for leafy greens and quick-cooking vegetables.

3. Pressure Cooking:

This method reduces cooking time, preserving heat-sensitive nutrients. It's excellent for legumes, whole grains, and tougher vegetable cuts.

4. Raw Preparation:

Consume some vegetables raw to maximize nutrient retention. Create salads, slaws, or use raw vegetables as crudités.

5. Proper Storage:

Store fruits and vegetables properly to maintain their nutrient content. Keep most produce in the refrigerator, but store tomatoes, potatoes, and onions in a cool, dark place.

6. Minimal Water Cooking:

When boiling, use minimal water and cook for the shortest time possible. Save the cooking liquid for soups or sauces to retain leached nutrients.

7. Gentle Reheating:

Reheat leftovers gently to prevent further nutrient loss. Use lower heat settings and add a splash of water if needed.

Time-saving Kitchen Hacks

1. Batch Cooking:

Prepare large quantities of staples like grains, legumes, and roasted vegetables to use throughout the week.

2. Freezer Meals:

Prepare and freeze individual portions of soups, stews, and casseroles for quick future meals.

3. One-Pan Meals:

Utilize sheet pan dinners or skillet meals to reduce prep time and cleanup.

4. Smart Chopping:

Invest in good knives and practice efficient chopping techniques. Pre-chop vegetables for multiple meals at once.

5. Instant Pot Utilization:

Use a multi-cooker like an Instant Pot for quick, hands-off cooking of grains, legumes, and proteins.

6. Microwave Shortcuts:

Use the microwave to quickly cook potatoes, steam vegetables, or melt ingredients for recipes.

7. Mise en Place:

Prepare all ingredients before starting to cook to streamline the cooking process.

8. Double Duty Cooking:

While preparing one meal, cook extra ingredients to use in future meals (e.g., roast extra vegetables or grill additional chicken).

Ingredient Substitutions

1. Egg Replacements:
- For binding: 1 tablespoon ground flaxseed mixed with 3 tablespoons water
- For moisture: ¼ cup mashed banana or applesauce
- For leavening: 1 teaspoon baking soda mixed with 1 tablespoon vinegar

2. Dairy Alternatives:
- Milk: Use unsweetened almond, soy, or oat milk
- Butter: Substitute with coconut oil or avocado in baking
- Cream: Use full-fat coconut milk or cashew cream

3. Flour Substitutions:
- All-purpose flour: Use almond flour or coconut flour for low-carb options
- Wheat flour: Substitute with spelt or oat flour for different nutritional profiles

4. Sugar Alternatives:
- Refined sugar: Use mashed dates, maple syrup, or stevia
- Brown sugar: Coconut sugar or date sugar can provide similar flavor

5. Oil Replacements:
- In baking: Replace oil with applesauce or Greek yogurt
- In cooking: Use vegetable broth for sautéing

6. Nut Substitutions:
- Tree nuts: Use seeds like pumpkin or sunflower seeds
- Peanut butter: Substitute with sunflower seed butter or tahini

7. Meat Alternatives:
- Ground meat: Use crumbled tempeh or textured vegetable protein
- Chicken: Substitute with firm tofu or seitan

8. Grain Swaps:
- Rice: Use cauliflower rice or quinoa
- Pasta: Try zucchini noodles or spaghetti squash

9. Soy Sauce Alternative:

Use coconut aminos for a soy-free, lower-sodium option

10. Breadcrumb Substitutes:

Use ground nuts, seeds, or rolled oats for a gluten-free coating

Chapter 10: Supplementing Your Diet

When it comes to supporting your hormonal health, the right supplements can play a valuable role in bridging any nutritional gaps in your diet. However, it's important to approach supplements with care and ensure you're making informed choices. In this chapter, we'll dive into the world of hormone-balancing supplements, provide guidance on selecting high-quality products, and discuss potential interactions with hormone replacement therapy (HRT).

Understanding Hormone-Balancing Supplements

The world of supplements can be overwhelming, with countless options claiming to support women's health. When it comes to maintaining hormonal balance, certain supplements have shown promise in clinical studies. Some of the most well-researched and widely recommended supplements for hormonal health include:

1. Omega-3 Fatty Acids: Found in fatty fish, walnuts, and flaxseeds, omega-3s have been shown to help reduce inflammation and support estrogen metabolism.

2. Vitamin D: This essential nutrient plays a crucial role in calcium absorption, bone health, and immune function – all of which are important for women's wellness.

3. Magnesium: Responsible for over 300 bodily processes, magnesium is particularly beneficial for managing stress, regulating sleep, and supporting reproductive health.

4. Black Cohosh: This herb has been used traditionally to help alleviate menopausal symptoms, such as hot flashes and night sweats.

5. Maca Root: Hailed as an adaptogen, maca may help balance hormones, boost energy, and improve mood during the menopausal transition.

6. Dong Quai: Also known as "female ginseng," this herb is believed to have a gentle, regulating effect on the female reproductive system.

It's important to note that the effectiveness and safety of supplements can vary, and they should not be viewed as a substitute for a well-balanced, nutrient-dense diet. Always consult with your healthcare provider before incorporating any new supplements into your routine, especially if you're currently taking HRT or other medications.

Choosing High-Quality Supplements

When selecting supplements to support your hormonal health, quality is paramount. Look for products from reputable brands that use third-party testing and certification, such as NSF International or USP. These organizations ensure supplements meet strict purity, potency, and safety standards.

When evaluating a supplement, consider the following factors:
- Ingredient list: Ensure the supplement contains the active ingredients you're seeking and that the formulation is free from unnecessary fillers or additives.
- Dosage: Check that the serving size aligns with the recommended intake for the specific nutrient or herb.
- Third-party testing: Look for the NSF, USP, or other trusted certification seals to verify the supplement's quality and purity.
- Company reputation: Research the manufacturer's track record and consumer reviews to gauge their commitment to producing high-quality products.

Potential Interactions with Hormone Replacement Therapy

If you're currently taking HRT, it's crucial to be mindful of potential interactions between your medication and any supplements you wish to incorporate. Some supplements, such as St. John's Wort, may interfere with the effectiveness of HRT, while others, like black cohosh, may provide complementary benefits.

Chapter 11: Exercise and Lifestyle for Hormonal Balance

Maintaining hormonal balance is a multifaceted endeavor, and your exercise routine and overall lifestyle choices play a crucial role in this delicate dance. In this chapter, we'll explore the best exercises for women's health, effective stress management techniques, and the profound importance of quality sleep – all essential components of the Estrogen Matters approach to holistic wellness.

Leveraging the Influence of Movement

When it comes to supporting your hormonal health, the right exercise regimen can be a game-changer. Physical activity not only helps manage weight and maintain muscle mass, but it also has a direct impact on the production and regulation of your key hormones.

Here are some of the most beneficial exercises for women seeking hormonal balance:

1. Strength Training: Lifting weights, whether with free weights or resistance bands, helps build and maintain lean muscle mass, which in turn supports healthy estrogen levels. Aim for 2-3 strength-training sessions per week, focusing on compound exercises that engage multiple muscle groups.

2. High-Intensity Interval Training (HIIT): Short bursts of intense exercise followed by periods of active recovery have been shown to boost insulin sensitivity, regulate cortisol (the stress hormone), and support overall hormonal balance. Incorporate HIIT workouts 1-2 times per week for maximum benefits.

3. Yoga and Pilates: These mind-body practices not only improve flexibility and core strength but also have a calming effect on the nervous system, helping to manage stress and reduce inflammation – both of which are crucial for hormonal equilibrium. Aim for 2-3 yoga or Pilates sessions per week.

4. Brisk Walking: Don't underestimate the power of a simple, yet effective, cardiovascular exercise like walking. Brisk walks, especially in nature, can help stabilize mood, reduce anxiety, and support healthy estrogen levels. Strive for 30-60 minutes of walking most days of the week.

When designing your exercise routine, be mindful of not overtraining, as excessive or intense physical activity can have the opposite effect and disrupt your hormonal balance. Listen to your body, and find a balanced approach that feels sustainable and empowering.

Mastering Stress Management

Stress is a silent saboteur when it comes to hormonal health. Chronic stress can lead to elevated cortisol levels, which can in turn disrupt the delicate dance of your other hormones, such as estrogen, progesterone, and thyroid hormones. Therefore, it's essential to prioritize effective stress management strategies as part of the Estrogen Matters lifestyle.

Here are some proven techniques to help you manage stress and support hormonal balance:

1. Meditation and Mindfulness: Dedicating just 10-15 minutes per day to a mindfulness practice, such as meditation, deep breathing, or guided visualization, can have a profound impact on your stress levels and overall sense of well-being.

2. Journaling: The act of putting pen to paper and expressing your thoughts, feelings, and emotions can be a powerful stress-relief tool. Experiment with different journaling styles, such as stream-of-consciousness writing or gratitude lists, to find what resonates most with you.

3. Gentle Movement: Low-impact activities like gentle yoga, Tai Chi, or leisurely walks can help calm the mind, reduce physical tension, and promote the release of feel-good hormones like endorphins.

4. Social Connection: Maintaining a healthy social support network, whether through regular meetups with friends, family gatherings, or joining a community group, can help mitigate the negative effects of stress on your hormonal balance.

5. Boundary Setting: Learning to say "no" to obligations or activities that deplete your energy can be a challenging but necessary skill. Prioritize self-care and create boundaries that allow you to recharge and maintain a state of equilibrium.

Remember, stress management is not a one-size-fits-all endeavor. Experiment with different techniques and find the combination that works best for your unique needs and lifestyle.

The Indispensable Role of Sleep

When it comes to hormonal health, the importance of quality sleep cannot be overstated. Your body's circadian rhythms, which govern the intricate dance of your hormones, are deeply influenced by the quantity and quality of your sleep. Disruptions to this delicate balance can have far-reaching consequences for your overall well-being.

Here's why sleep is so critical for hormonal balance:
1. Melatonin Production: Melatonin, often referred to as the "sleep hormone," plays a crucial role in regulating your body's sleep-wake cycle. Adequate melatonin production not only helps you fall and stay asleep but also supports the proper functioning of other hormones, such as estrogen and testosterone.

2. Cortisol Regulation: As mentioned earlier, chronic stress and elevated cortisol levels can wreak havoc on your hormonal balance. Quality sleep helps keep cortisol in check, allowing your body to better manage stress and maintain hormonal equilibrium.

3. Growth Hormone Release: During deep, restorative sleep, your body releases growth hormone, which is essential for tissue repair, muscle growth, and the maintenance of healthy bone density – all of which are important for women's overall health and wellness.

4. Insulin Sensitivity: Poor sleep has been linked to decreased insulin sensitivity, which can lead to imbalances in blood sugar regulation and potentially contribute to conditions like polycystic ovary syndrome (PCOS) and metabolic disorders.

To ensure your sleep supports your hormonal health, aim for 7-9 hours of quality sleep each night. Establish a consistent sleep routine, create a sleep-conducive environment, and consider incorporating relaxation techniques, such as gentle stretching or meditation, into your pre-bedtime rituals.

Embracing the Estrogen Matters Lifestyle

By incorporating regular exercise, effective stress management, and quality sleep into your daily life, you'll be taking a significant step towards supporting your hormonal balance and overall well-being. Remember, this is a journey, and finding the right balance may require some trial and error. Be patient, listen to your body, and celebrate the small victories along the way.

As you continue to explore the Estrogen Matters approach, remember that your health and happiness are the ultimate priorities. Embrace the power of mindful self-care, and trust that by nourishing your body, mind, and spirit, you'll unlock the key to a vibrant, hormonally balanced life.

CONCLUSION

As we reach the end of our exploration of the Estrogen Matters approach, it's important to reflect on the transformative power of this holistic methodology. Throughout this comprehensive guide, we've delved into the intricate world of women's hormonal health, uncovering the profound connections between estrogen, thyroid function, and overall well-being. From understanding the nuances of hormone replacement therapy to embracing the restorative benefits of exercise, stress management, and quality sleep, we've armed you with the knowledge and tools to take charge of your hormonal health and unlock a vibrant, energized future.

Remember, your journey towards hormonal balance is a deeply personal one, and the path forward may look different for each individual. But by embracing the Estrogen Matters principles, you'll be empowered to make informed decisions that align with your unique needs and preferences. Whether it's working closely with a trusted healthcare provider to optimize your hormone levels, or implementing lifestyle changes that nourish your mind, body, and spirit, the choice is yours. Trust your intuition, listen to your body, and don't be afraid to advocate for your health – for it is the foundation upon which you will build a life of boundless energy, resilience, and joy.

As you continue to navigate the complexities of hormonal health, remember that you are not alone. The Estrogen Matters community is here to support you every step of the way, offering a wealth of resources, including expert-curated content, informative webinars, and a vibrant online forum where you can connect with like-minded individuals. Embrace the power of knowledge, collaboration, and mutual understanding, for it is through these connections that we will collectively transform the narrative around women's health and empower a new generation of thriving, hormonally balanced individuals.

So, as you close this chapter and embark on the next leg of your empowering health journey, remember to celebrate your progress, embrace the challenges, and continue to seek out the information and support that will guide you towards optimal well-being. Your hormonal health is a precious gift, and by nurturing it with intention and care, you'll unlock the key to a life brimming with vitality, resilience, and boundless possibilities.

We invite you to share your feedback, insights, and personal experiences with us. Your reviews and ratings will not only help us improve the Estrogen Matters resource but also inspire and uplift others who are on a similar path of self-discovery and empowerment. Together, let's continue to redefine the narrative around women's health and create a future where hormonal balance is the norm, not the exception.